First Aid for Motorists

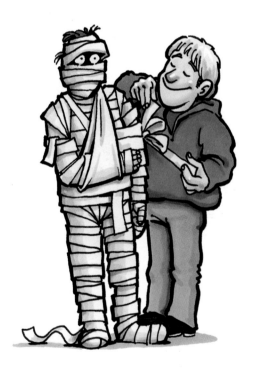

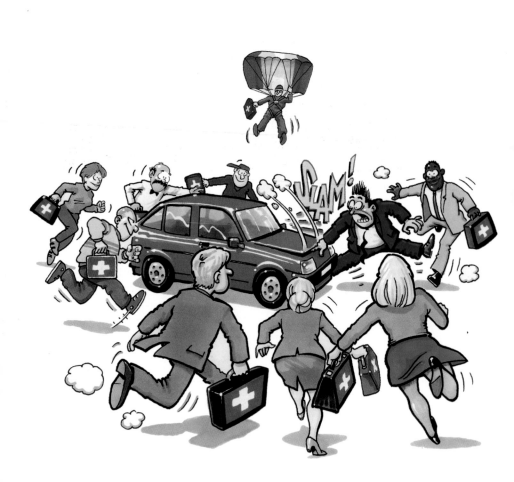

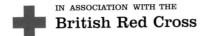

IN ASSOCIATION WITH THE
British Red Cross

First Aid for Motorists

Published by
the British School of Motoring Ltd.
in association with Virgin Publishing

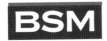

Virgin

First published in the UK in 1997 by
The British School of Motoring Ltd
81/87 Hartfield Road
Wimbledon
LONDON SW19 3TJ

The Hazchem signs contained in this book are reproduced by the kind permission
of Her Majesty's Stationery Office.

ISBN 0 7535 0135 X

Written by Anita Eade

Cartoons by Marc Lacey
of The Visual Works

Photographs by Steve Gorton

Illustrations by Oliver Frey

Design, typesetting and reprographics by Prima Creative Services

Printed in Germany by Neue Stalling

The publishers would like to thank the staff and friends from BSM and
the British Red Cross who helped with the photography for this book.

Please note: The red cross emblem is an international sign of protection during armed conflict,
and its use is restricted by law. The European Union symbol for first aid is a white cross on a green background.

The use of the Red Cross name and emblem does not in any way suggest an endorsement of a company
or its products or services.

Contents

Why a Book on First Aid?

THE MULTITUDE OF BRITISH AND American hospital dramas, coupled with the trend for shows reconstructing accidents, have brought dramatic first aid scenes into our living rooms. Think back to any of these shows, and I guarantee that one of the incidents you will remember will involve a motorist of some description. This is not because car scenes are cheaper to film than any others but is a true reflection of the many accidents that take place on British roads every year. Combine a metal box moving at 30mph with trees, bridges and other immovable objects, sprinkle in bad weather conditions, other road users and poor visibility, and you have a recipe for potential disaster.

This said, it is not all doom and gloom for the motorist. Of the 310,000 road accidents involving casualties yearly, most do not involve major injury to the participants. However, of those that do, the actions of the first to arrive on the scene will often have a dramatic effect on the outcome of the incident.

Who is usually the first person to arrive at the scene of a car accident? Ideally it would be someone from one of the emergency services, but the reality is usually otherwise.

The person in a position to offer immediate life-saving help at the scene of an accident is most likely to be you – the next motorist to drive along the road.

And that is where *First Aid for Motorists* comes in. This book doesn't claim it can turn you into a paramedic, nurse or doctor, but it does aim to start you on the road towards keeping the casualty alive long enough for experts to do their stuff. The best doctor in the world can do little with the casualty who is dead on arrival.

Happening on an accident is always frightening – even experienced paramedics never know what to expect – but preparation is everything. First aid needs minimal equipment – you can do most things just with your hands, breath and voice – but it does require a cool head, a knowledge of what to do and, just as importantly, what not to do.

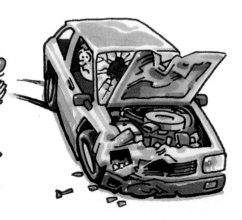

PRACTISING YOUR FIRST AID SKILLS

First aid is a very practical subject. Although this book is an excellent guide to the life-saving skills you need to know but hope you will never have to use, it cannot be a substitute for first aid training. The British Red Cross runs a range of courses to suit every individual, including one specifically aimed at motorists. For details of the courses nearest to you, contact your local Branch Headquarters listed in the telephone directory under British Red Cross.

HOW TO USE THIS BOOK

First Aid for Motorists is written in a very informal way. Although I shall talk to you as 'I', this book – like others in the BSM series – reflects the collected knowledge of experts in the field. Throughout, I have tried to give you examples of real-life incidents that demonstrate the importance of effective first aid. The book also relies heavily on the use of photographs, drawings, cartoons and key points to reinforce the essential elements of first aid and of the action to be taken at a road accident.

While I hope that you will have a chance to read the contents before you need to use any of the knowledge gained, you may come across an accident on the way home. In which case *First Aid for Motorists'* EMERGENCY INDEX will quickly enable you to find the key information that you will require.

I hope that this book is one you will refer to on a regular basis, as first aid skills need to be kept up to date. I would suggest that you keep it in the glove compartment or boot of your car along with your first aid kit, blanket and hazard warning triangle. You mean you haven't got these things in your car – then read on...

Anita Eade

Anita Eade BA (Hons) QTS is the First Aid Training Manager for the British Red Cross

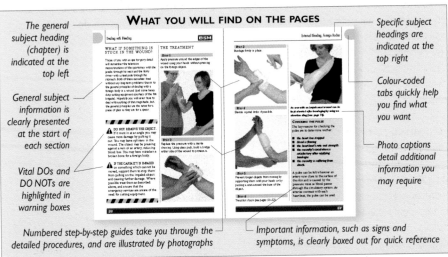

WHAT YOU WILL FIND ON THE PAGES

The general subject heading (chapter) is indicated at the top left

General subject information is clearly presented at the start of each section

Vital DOs and DO NOTs are highlighted in warning boxes

Specific subject headings are indicated at the top right

Colour-coded tabs quickly help you find what you want

Photo captions detail additional information you may require

Numbered step-by-step guides take you through the detailed procedures, and are illustrated by photographs

Important information, such as signs and symptoms, is clearly boxed out for quick reference

What is First Aid?

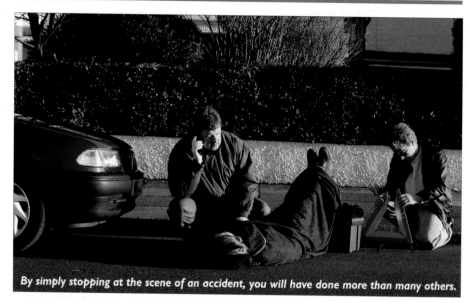

By simply stopping at the scene of an accident, you will have done more than many others.

A S ITS NAME SUGGESTS, FIRST AID is the first help given to a person who has been injured, or who suddenly becomes ill, before 'second aid' arrives. We will discuss this notion of second aid later, but generally at road accidents it will be in the form of an ambulance – one of the few times a motorist is pleased to see a blue light coming up behind them.

Reading *First Aid for Motorists* will give you the underpinning knowledge to carry out first aid, but you should always remember that the term 'first aider' is generally applied to a person who has completed a set standard of training with an organization such as the British Red Cross Society.

First aid has three key aims, set out in the box below, which I will keep coming back to throughout this book when we start to look at the more detailed treatments for specific injuries and conditions.

FIRST AID'S THREE KEY AIMS

1. **To keep the casualty alive**

2. **To stop them getting worse**

3. **To promote their recovery**

LOOKING AFTER NUMBER ONE

One theme I will be emphasising time and again is the importance of keeping the first aider safe at the scene of an emergency. It is just as important to take care of yourself after the accident.

First aid, by its very nature, is often a highly emotional activity and it is important that you have the chance to discuss how you feel after helping at the scene of an accident. Talk to your friends and family about what happened, what you did and how you feel.

Should you want to discuss the incident in more depth, contact your local British Red Cross Branch who will be able to advise you on other areas of support. Remember, though, that by simply stopping at an accident you will have done much more than many others, and whatever the outcome of the incident, you deserve to congratulate yourself for that.

FIRST AID EQUIPMENT

Most first aid procedures can be carried out without special equipment. However, there is no harm in carrying a few helpful bits and pieces.

Possibly the most important thing to do at the scene of an accident is to keep the area around the incident safe. Many car accidents are added to by the next vehicle whizzing around the bend. The best way to keep safe is with a hazard warning triangle. Most European countries insist on drivers carrying one in the vehicle, and they are recognised internationally as the symbol of trouble ahead. All good garages carry them, and they are not an expensive item.

Another key need at the accident scene is to keep the victims warm – either those seriously hurt or those wandering around in an upset state. Keeping one or two blankets in the boot of your car will take up little space and could be potentially life-saving.

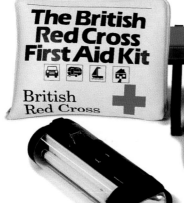

Make sure you always carry a hazard warning triangle, a working torch and some blankets in addition to your first aid kit.

THE FIRST AID KIT

There are many first aid kits available on the market, but I recommend that you purchase a soft kit; either that or fasten your kit down in the glove compartment. The least number of things that you have flying about inside the car, the less your personal risk of head injury should you be forced to brake suddenly.

As a guide, a first aid kit should at least contain the following:

- disposable gloves
- a number of triangular bandages
- a large sterile dressing for treating major bleeding or burns
- plasters for smaller cuts and grazes, and alcohol-free wipes with which to clean smaller wounds.

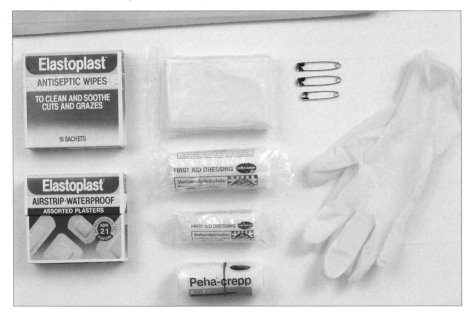

⚠ FIRST AID EQUIPMENT like this should be available at any good chemist. If you have any problems getting the equipment, contact your local British Red Cross, who will be able to provide you with what you need at a reasonable price.

Other useful items would include:

- plastic sandwich, or freezer bags for enclosing dressed hand or arm burns
- some safety pins for fastening bandages
- a small pair of round-nosed scissors for trimming bandages or cutting away clothing making a wound inaccessible
- water for cooling burns and for making cold compresses.

Action at an Emergency

THE FIRST AND MOST OBVIOUS PIECE of advice is 'don't panic!'. While this may appear easier said than done, there are a few simple things you can do to help calm yourself down. Many of these are general rules, which should be applied at the scene of any accident – whether it be a ten-car crash or a cyclist with a grazed knee. This chapter looks at these rules and considers the importance of safety at every accident scene you may come across.

ON COMING ACROSS AN ACCIDENT

At any accident scene remember to take a deep breath, and do not rush. If you are on foot, walk up to the accident – don't run.

Combining panic with exertion leaves most of us out of breath, and taking charge of a car crash between gasps for air will hardly inspire confidence in your leadership qualities – never mind leaving you fit enough to give a casualty mouth-to-mouth resuscitation.

If you are in a car, remember to check your mirrors and pull up safely behind the incident. Make sure that you and your car are visible and that the accident scene is protected from oncoming drivers. One of the best ways of ensuring that your car can be seen is to use your hazard lights. Only apply them, however, when you are stationary; using them while moving may leave any car following second-guessing as to what you are going to do.

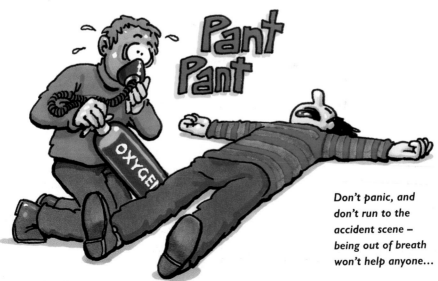

Don't panic, and don't run to the accident scene – being out of breath won't help anyone...

PERSONAL SAFETY – CHECKING FOR DANGER

The first rule at any emergency is always, always **CHECK FOR DANGER!**

As the first aider, you are the most important person to arrive at an emergency scene. After all, without you, lifesaving procedures won't be carried out and the emergency services won't be called. Hurting yourself rules out a lifeline for everybody else – don't do it.

ONCOMING TRAFFIC

The most obvious danger is oncoming traffic. Think before you step out onto the road yourself. Can you be seen? Can your car be seen? Can the accident be seen? I have mentioned parking behind the accident to protect the scene of the crash, but on sharp bends or with poor visibility further action might be necessary.

If the accident is on a bend, try to set up some warning for other drivers; the ideal item is the hazard warning triangle. Additionally bystanders can flag down traffic if it is safe for them to do so. If you are on the road or even the roadside, ensure that you can be seen.

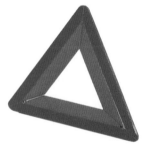

A hazard warning triangle can be bought from all good garages and motoring shops.

High-visibility strips are the best source of protection, but alternatively take off dark coats or outer clothes.

If the accident is on a busy road or a motorway, it is unlikely that you will be able to stop safely. Drive past the accident to the nearest telephone and call for help.

FIRE

If a car is going to catch fire, it will generally do so on impact. But contrary to popular film fiction, the slightest impact does not cause most cars to burst into flames. However, there is always a danger of fire at any road accident. To reduce the risk:

- ensure nobody smokes around the accident site
- ensure the ignition of any involved vehicle is switched off
- if possible, isolate the battery
- if possible, cover petrol spills with earth, and keep bystanders well away from the scene of the accident.

WHAT IF A CAR IS ON FIRE? If there are people trapped in a burning car do not attempt to rescue them yourself – call the fire brigade, and get everybody back from the accident scene. Do not attempt to fight the fire yourself.

BROKEN GLASS AND METAL

Broken glass and twisted metal are real dangers to first aiders at the site of a crash and care should be taken to avoid cutting yourself as you move in or around a car.

UNSECURED VEHICLES

I once found myself rolling down a hill in a car after a minor accident because both the other driver and myself (not unreasonably, considering our circumstances) had failed to put on our handbrakes. I had no excuse, and was lucky that the most I suffered was a red face. Before getting into a car ensure that it is not going to move any further – if necessary, put blocks under the wheels, and if in doubt, don't get in.

SUMMARY

■ Protect the scene and yourself from oncoming traffic

■ Take steps to further reduce the risk of fire

■ Ensure that the car is stable before getting into it

■ Take care not to cut yourself on glass or metal

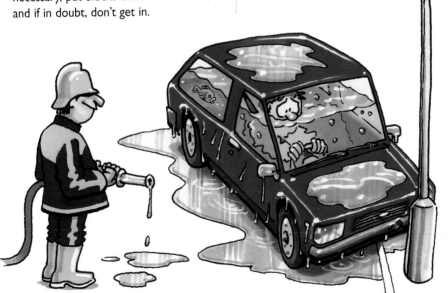

If your own car catches fire while driving, stop, get everybody out and call the fire brigade. Do not attempt to fight the fire yourself.

MAKING AN ASSESSMENT, GETTING HELP

After checking for danger the second rule is to make an assessment of the incident.

The first thing to assess is the number of people involved. In a large accident the total number may be difficult to ascertain, but it is important to be aware of potential hidden casualties: the pillion motorcyclist, the baby in the back of the car, the passenger who may have wandered away from the scene confused.

The next thing you need to determine is who are the most seriously injured. Although disconcerting, the screaming casualty is not generally in immediate danger of dying, whereas the quiet casualty may be suffering from a blocked airway, breathing difficulties or circulatory problems that may prove fatal if not treated promptly. The importance of the ABC of first aid is discussed in more detail on pages 17–30.

CALLING FOR HELP

Once you have ascertained the number of casualties and treated any life-threatening conditions, the next rule is to call for appropriate help. Of course, another bystander may have already done so, but it is vital to make sure that the call to the emergency services has actually been placed by someone.

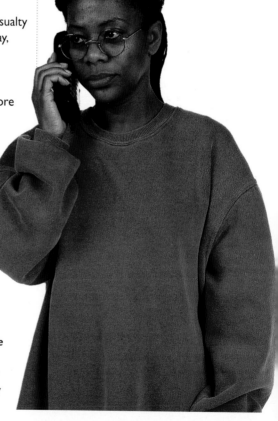

For the professional first aider, a mobile phone may be a necessity rather than a luxury, since you never know how far away the nearest public telephone may be, especially in more isolated areas.

THE 999 CALL

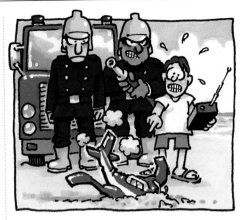

Many calls the emergency services receive fail to provide them with the appropriate information. Surely none, however, could surpass a call that a colleague of mine received on his first day in control of a local fire station. On being told that a plane had crashed into a crowded beach, he sent three fire engines and put out a call for back-up. Imagine his dismay (relief?) on finding that the plane was a two-seater whose pilot and passenger had crash-landed on an empty part of the beach and then walked away from the accident with only minor injuries. The moral of the story is to make your message clear.

DIAL 999

- If in doubt about which emergency services you require, call the police who will contact the appropriate help.
- You will be asked for your name. Generally, the operator can tell which number you are calling from, but if not, you may be asked for this.
- Give details of exactly where the accident is. A common mistake is to give the address as the 'High Street' – have you any idea how many High Streets there are in Britain?
- Try to identify landmarks, junction numbers or even house numbers in a residential area – this reduces the time that the emergency services have to spend looking for you.
- If you are in an area that is difficult to reach, such as an industrial site, it is often a good idea to agree to send somebody to meet the emergency services at an easily identifiable location – perhaps the site entrance.
- Give a description of the accident scene and identify any particular hazards or points of note, for example trapped casualties or chemicals (*see page 16*). Each Fire Brigade tends to have specialist equipment located at different stations, so the sooner they are aware of specific problems, the sooner they can call for the appropriate back-up.
- Tell the emergency services how many casualties you believe there are and give at least an idea of what injuries there appear to be.
- Do not hang up until the operator tells you to.

ONGOING ACTION AT AN EMERGENCY

You will need to continue giving first aid care to casualties according to the priority that their injuries accord them. Airway, breathing and circulatory problems (such as heart failure and major bleeding) must always come first. Where possible, it is essential to keep casualties still after any accident, particularly when there has been any sudden impact or deceleration. The risk of neck injuries is ever present. Accident victims who showed no apparent injuries at the time of an accident have often been diagnosed as suffering from whiplash or neck fractures some time later. These problems are dealt with in more detail on pages 71–74.

Remember to ask if there is anybody else around who knows first aid, as people may be unwilling to come forward unless asked. And always accept help if it is to hand; don't end up in the situation a colleague of mine found himself in. He was busily dealing with a casualty suffering from a major bleed and kept brushing off the attentions of a woman who was offering to help. Eventually she lost all patience and told him that when he got to the bit about calling for the doctor, she was already there!

In a larger accident you may have to use others to reassure the less seriously injured casualties, or upset bystanders, relatives or friends. It doesn't take a lot of first aid knowledge to reassure an upset onlooker or to keep somebody warm, yet these are two of the vital steps in treating an accident victim for shock (see pages 49–52), a potentially fatal condition.

It is important not to get in the way of ambulance crews, doctors, police or fire officers, but equally you will often have information that can help all three services. Advise the crews that you have been on the scene and offer responses to any questions they may have. For example, it is important for the ambulance crew to know if an unconscious casualty has been unconscious since the crash or whether their condition has deteriorated since the accident occurred.

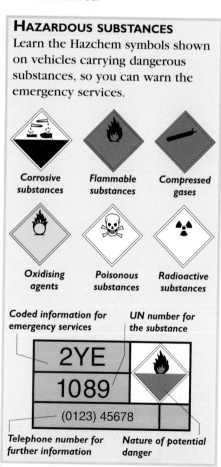

HAZARDOUS SUBSTANCES
Learn the Hazchem symbols shown on vehicles carrying dangerous substances, so you can warn the emergency services.

Corrosive substances

Flammable substances

Compressed gases

Oxidising agents

Poisonous substances

Radioactive substances

Coded information for emergency services

UN number for the substance

2YE

1089

(0123) 45678

Telephone number for further information

Nature of potential danger

Dealing with Unconsciousness

WHILE THE CASUALTY WHO SCREAMS and shouts is very distressing to see and hear, the casualty who makes little or no noise is often the one most at risk of dying. The quiet casualty may be unconscious, and any unconscious casualty is likely to be suffering from some degree of airway difficulties.

This chapter introduces you to the

ABC

(Airway, Breathing and Circulation)
of first aid, and shows you the simple manoeuvres which could save the life of an unconscious casualty.

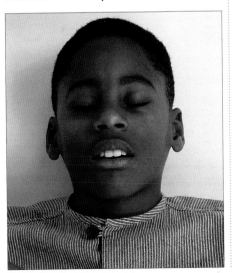

WHAT IS UNCONSCIOUSNESS?

Unconsciousness can be described as a lack of normal brain activity – there is a loss of response to stimuli and a loss of awareness.

While the cause may not be of prime importance for the first aider, it is useful to know the more common causes because the first aider may have a chance to identify signs and symptoms that will provide useful information to the ambulance crew.

Among the most common causes are those listed in the box below. All of these causes are described in more detail in their respective chapters of this book, together with an outline of the signs and symptoms that a first aider should look for, and the treatment for the specific problems.

Head injury *(see page 61)*
Heart attack/stroke *(see pages 105-106/110)*
Epilepsy *(see pages 108-109)*
Temperature extremes *(see pages 95-96)*
Lack of oxygen *(see pages 19-20)*
Fainting *(see page 30)*
Shock *(see pages 49-52)*

WHATEVER THE CAUSE, the treatment of any unconscious casualty always follows the same set of rules.

ASSESSING AN UNCONSCIOUS CASUALTY

The most important first action with any casualty is to check for danger. And this remains your priority even if you suspect that one or more of the casualties is unconscious.

Having checked for danger, the next step is to assess the scene by using the rule that the quietest casualty is often the one most at risk.

Having found a casualty that you believe may be unconscious, you must check to see if they really are. I know of a friend who was in the embarrassing situation of being slapped by a sunbather he thought was unconscious. In fact she was only having a snooze on the beach. I can't help but feel that he was a little too eager to try mouth to mouth resuscitation...

CHECKING FOR CONSCIOUSNESS

■ *Talk to the casualty on approaching them. Kneel down next to them and ask them a question to try and provoke a response.*

■ *Gently shake the casualty by the shoulders (be gentle as there may be the risk of neck injuries).*

■ *If there is no response to this, assume that the casualty is unconscious.*

We will consider the various degrees of impaired awareness later on in this chapter, but for now it is enough to know that a lack of response means that this casualty is in danger of dying if their airway isn't protected.

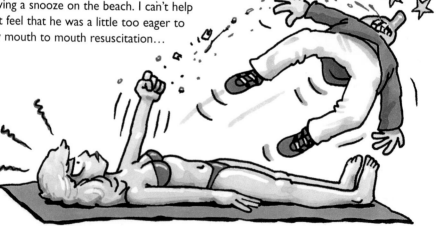

AIRWAY

Having ascertained that a casualty actually *is* unconscious, the priority now is to check and maintain an open airway.

WHAT IS THE AIRWAY?

The airway can be described as the passage from the nose and mouth, down the trachea (windpipe) into the lungs. To breathe effectively all these passages need to be clear and the other elements of the respiratory system need to be functioning adequately. These other elements include the ribs, which must be free to move out (breathing in) and move in (breathing out), the diaphragm and adequate oxygen.

WHY DO WE NEED AN OPEN AIRWAY?

The body needs an open airway to allow an adequate supply of oxygen into the circulatory system. The circulatory system carries the blood to all the body's tissues and organs (see also *Dealing with Bleeding, pages 53–62*). With insufficient oxygen to the vital organs, particularly the brain, the body will shut down, and death will eventually result.

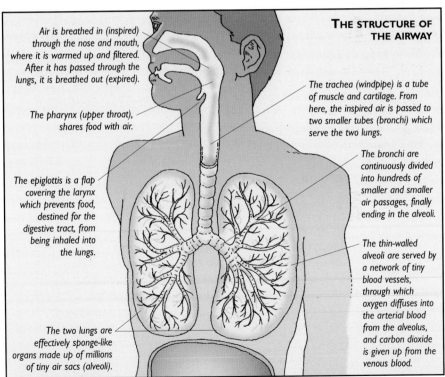

THE STRUCTURE OF THE AIRWAY

Air is breathed in (inspired) through the nose and mouth, where it is warmed up and filtered. After it has passed through the lungs, it is breathed out (expired).

The pharynx (upper throat), shares food with air.

The epiglottis is a flap covering the larynx which prevents food, destined for the digestive tract, from being inhaled into the lungs.

The two lungs are effectively sponge-like organs made up of millions of tiny air sacs (alveoli).

The trachea (windpipe) is a tube of muscle and cartilage. From here, the inspired air is passed to two smaller tubes (bronchi) which serve the two lungs.

The bronchi are continuously divided into hundreds of smaller and smaller air passages, finally ending in the alveoli.

The thin-walled alveoli are served by a network of tiny blood vessels, through which oxygen diffuses into the arterial blood from the alveolus, and carbon dioxide is given up from the venous blood.

THE BREATHING PROCESS

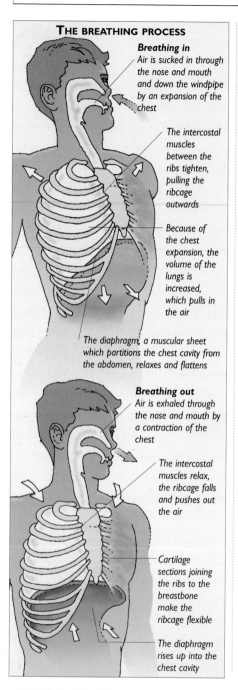

Breathing in
Air is sucked in through the nose and mouth and down the windpipe by an expansion of the chest

The intercostal muscles between the ribs tighten, pulling the ribcage outwards

Because of the chest expansion, the volume of the lungs is increased, which pulls in the air

The diaphragm, a muscular sheet which partitions the chest cavity from the abdomen, relaxes and flattens

Breathing out
Air is exhaled through the nose and mouth by a contraction of the chest

The intercostal muscles relax, the ribcage falls and pushes out the air

Cartilage sections joining the ribs to the breastbone make the ribcage flexible

The diaphragm rises up into the chest cavity

MAKING A CLEAR AIRWAY

Your first task is to remove any potential obstructions to the airway, such as a rope around the neck or a heavy object on the chest preventing the ribs rising, etc.

If you are unable to remove any restrictions to breathing – perhaps the object on the chest is too heavy, or the casualty is in a fume-filled environment that is too dangerous for you to enter – then call for help immediately.

THE DANGER OF CHOKING

The most common airway restriction is choking: that is, something actually blocking the air passages. The treatment for choking is covered in detail on pages 32–36, however, the priority *now* is to consider how to ensure that the unconscious casualty does not choke. The three things most likely to choke an unconscious casualty are:

- Tongue
- Sick
- Blood
  or TSB for short.

The tongue is a muscle, and in an unconscious state all the muscles relax and go floppy. With an unconscious casualty lying on their back the tongue slips to the back of the throat and blocks the airway.

There is a simple remedy for this that would save hundreds of lives every year if applied to unconscious casualties. If you remember nothing else from this book remember this!

OPENING THE AIRWAY

To open the airway place two fingers under the chin and lift the jaw. Place your other hand on the forehead and gently tilt the head backwards. This will stop the tongue from resting on the back of the throat and will maintain an open airway

This procedure can be carried out on an unconscious casualty sitting in a car to good effect by using the hands to support the neck and gently extending the airway by tilting the head back.

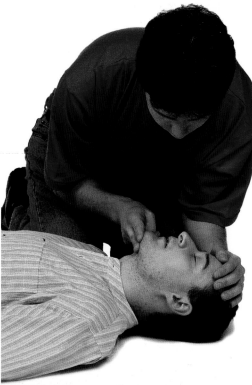

WHILE YOU SHOULD have an awareness of potential neck injuries, the protection of the airway always takes preference to the treatment of any potential condition.

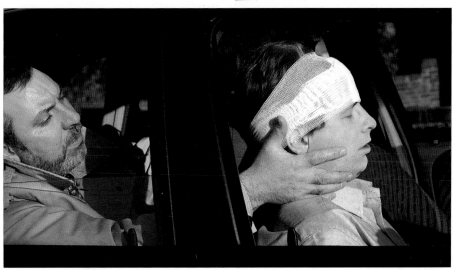

BREATHING

The next step in the ABC of first aid, having opened the airway, is to ascertain whether or not the casualty is breathing. In a quiet room, with the lights on, and the casualty lying flat on their back, checking to tell if they are breathing is relatively easy.

Murphy's Law of First Aid, however, states that your casualty is bound to be lying on their stomach beside the A1, in the pitch black, and in pouring rain. For this reason we have three checks to carry out to determine if a casualty is breathing.

> ### THREE BREATHING CHECKS
> 1. Look
> 2. Listen
> 3. Feel

What to do if the casualty is not breathing is dealt with in the resuscitation chapter on pages 39–47.

For now I shall look at the care of the casualty who *is* breathing and the steps you must take to ensure that they keep breathing until they either fully recover or can be moved to proper medical facilities.

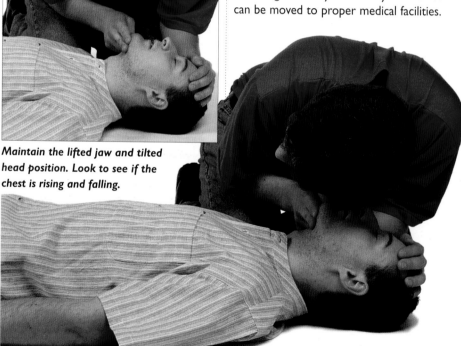

Maintain the lifted jaw and tilted head position. Look to see if the chest is rising and falling.

Listen for the sounds of breathing with your cheek by the side of the casualty's mouth.

Feel the casualty's breaths on your cheek.

THE RECOVERY POSITION

Lifting the jaw and tilting the head (*as covered on page 21*) will prevent the casualty from choking on their tongue. The next potential problem is the ever-present risk of vomiting.

As already stated, in an unconscious person all their muscles are relaxed. Because of this, there is also nothing holding in the contents of their stomach, so the casualty is likely to vomit. And if they are left on their back, there is a serious risk of the casualty choking on their own vomit. So the casualty needs to be moved into a position which minimises this risk while they are allowed to recover.

If they are in a position which already provides the four key factors shown in the box to the right, you need do no more than leave the casualty where they are and monitor their breathing and circulation.

If the position that they are in does not provide these four factors, you will have to move the casualty into the recovery position. It is unlikely that they will be lying flat on their back – as is shown in the following steps on pages 24–25 – but the procedures can be adapted to put the casualty into the recovery position however they are when you find them.

THE RECOVERY POSITION takes priority over most other conditions. If you suspect spinal injury or other fractures, the position can be modified as described on page 26. If the casualty has any life-threatening conditions, such as severe external bleeding, treat this first. If not, move the casualty straight into the recovery position.

RECOVERY POSITION

The recovery position gives the casualty:

- *a clear airway with no risk of obstruction by the tongue because the head is tilted back*

- *opportunity for blood and vomit to drain from the mouth because of the relative positions of the mouth to the airway*

- *room to breathe by ensuring that their chest is off the ground*

- *a stable position*

BSM

STEP 1
Ensure that their jaw is lifted and that their head is back.

STEP 2
Place the arm nearest you underneath the body with the fingers flat, palm upwards and the elbow straight.

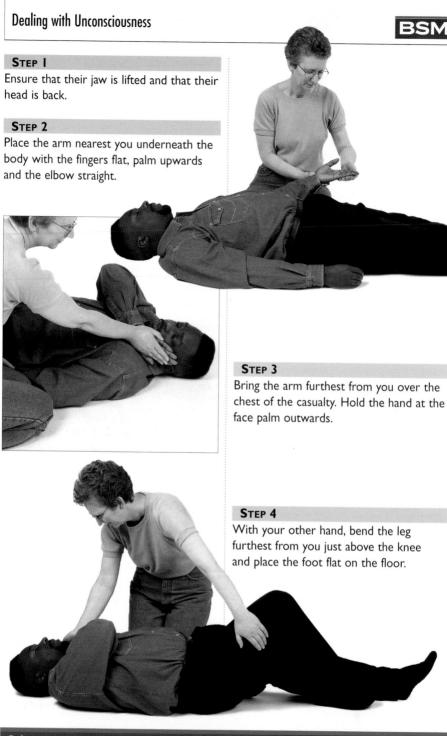

STEP 3
Bring the arm furthest from you over the chest of the casualty. Hold the hand at the face palm outwards.

STEP 4
With your other hand, bend the leg furthest from you just above the knee and place the foot flat on the floor.

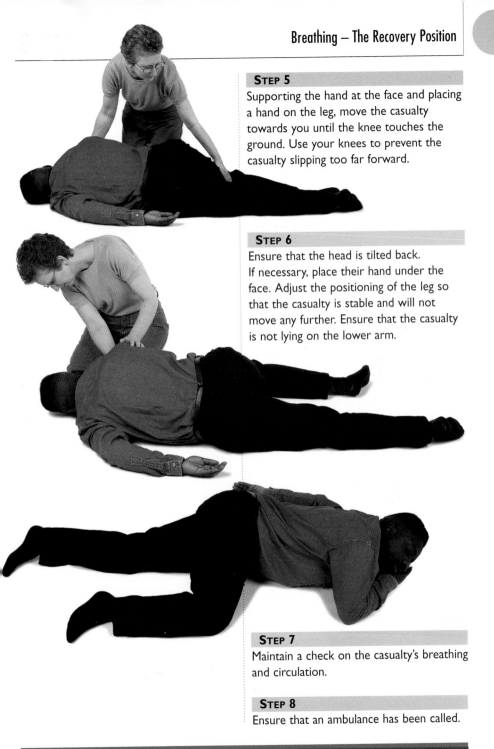

STEP 5

Supporting the hand at the face and placing a hand on the leg, move the casualty towards you until the knee touches the ground. Use your knees to prevent the casualty slipping too far forward.

STEP 6

Ensure that the head is tilted back. If necessary, place their hand under the face. Adjust the positioning of the leg so that the casualty is stable and will not move any further. Ensure that the casualty is not lying on the lower arm.

STEP 7

Maintain a check on the casualty's breathing and circulation.

STEP 8

Ensure that an ambulance has been called.

SPINAL INJURY RECOVERY POSITION

If you suspect that the casualty has a spinal injury, you still need to turn them into the recovery position. However, it is of particular importance to make sure that you reduce the risk of further damage to the spine.

If you have been trained to do so, move the head into the neutral position, if it is not already there.

This leaves the head in line with the neck and the spine. The nose should be in line with the navel. Ideally you will need the help of at least one bystander to turn the casualty into the recovery position.

STEP I

One person supports the head by firmly placing their hands over the casualty's ears. It is their responsibility to keep the head in line with the neck and spine and reduce the movement of the head from side to side, as shown above.

STEP 2

The second person prepares for the recovery position as shown previously in steps 1–4 on page 24.

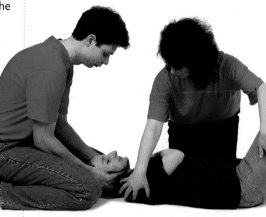

STEP 3

Move the casualty slowly over onto their side, keeping the head in line with the body, as shown below.

STEP 4

Once the casualty is on their side, the head should still be supported. If possible, the second first aider should continue to support the body.

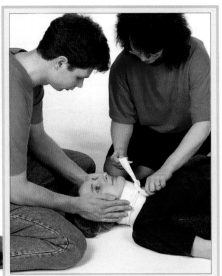

If you suspect a neck injury, a collar can be applied for additional support before turning.

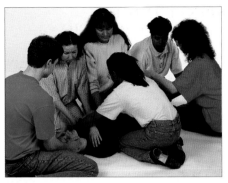

If you suspect that the casualty has suffered multiple fractures, you may have to enlist the help of up to five bystanders to turn the casualty into the recovery position.

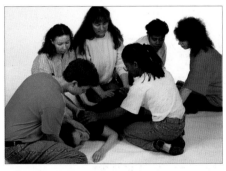

ALTERING THE RECOVERY POSITION

If you suspect that the casualty has fractures, you should ensure that the fracture is supported when turning the casualty. If it is difficult to bend an arm or leg because you suspect that it may be broken, keep it straight and use rolled up coats or blankets as props to ensure that the casualty stays on their side. However, always remember that if a casualty is breathing well and is already on their side with their head extended, they are often best left where they are.

THE PRIORITY with the unconscious casualty remains Airway and Breathing – maintain a constant check on the casualty's breathing and be prepared to resuscitate if it stops (*see Resuscitation, pages 39-46*). If they have time, the first aider may carry out a number of checks that might provide useful information to the ambulance service.

CIRCULATION

Circulation is the third component of the ABC of first aid – Airway, Breathing, Circulation.

The circulation – which simply describes the flow of blood around the body – can be checked by taking the pulse and looking for other signs of blood flow around the body, for example, skin colour, warm skin, capillary refill (see page 54).

If the casualty is breathing, they will have a pulse – the beat of the heart felt as a physical surge, or pulse, in the arteries – and some degree of circulation.

It is useful to know the rate, strength and rhythm of the pulse. This will provide a guide to the casualty's state, and possibly even a clue to the reason for their unconsciousness.

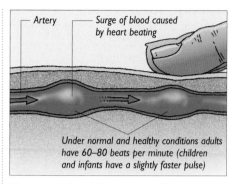

Artery — *Surge of blood caused by heart beating*

Under normal and healthy conditions adults have 60–80 beats per minute (children and infants have a slightly faster pulse)

The surge of each heartbeat is felt as a pulse from the artery under the finger.

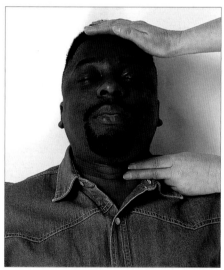

The pulse is best taken in the neck – at the carotid artery. Use two fingers and feel for the pulse in the groove to the side of the Adam's apple.

CHECKING THE CIRCULATION

■ Record the rate of the pulse, its strength and the rhythm.

■ Keep checking every five minutes and pass the information to the ambulance service.

■ If the pulse is very quick and continues getting quicker and weaker, it is possible that the casualty is suffering from shock. Check for any external bleeding that you may have missed, and treat the casualty for shock (see pages 49-52) in the hope of preventing further deterioration.

■ If you cannot feel a carotid pulse and the casualty is not breathing, commence CPR (see pages 39-47).

BODY CHECK

It is unlikely that you will have time to carry out an in-depth body check before the ambulance arrives. However, there are a number of key points to look for which may give you additional information for the ambulance crew and which may alter the treatment that you give the casualty.

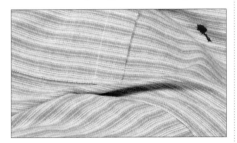

Check for bleeding – examine the casualty's clothes from top to toe to check for any damp patches. Dark, thick clothes absorb a great deal of blood, so a life-threatening severe bleed may not be immediately apparent.

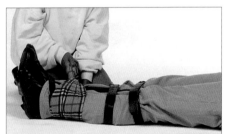

Check for fractures – look for swelling or deformity. If present, suspect a fracture, and provide extra padding and support around that area.

Check face colour and temperature – if the face is very pale, cold and clammy, this may indicate shock and/or a potential internal bleed.

LEVELS OF CONSCIOUSNESS

There are four levels of impaired awareness, described by the mnemonic:

AVPU

(Alert, Responds to Voice, Responds to Pain, Unresponsive)

We are generally in the alert state. Even when asleep, it takes little to make us alert.

A casualty may appear to be unconscious but may respond when asked a question, even if only with a grunt or a few words.

If a casualty has an injury, they may respond to pain, even though they do not respond to your voice. This response may be verbal but is more likely to be in the form of a grimace or twitch of the injured part. For this reason it is important to watch the casualty's face when treating an unconscious person since it may give you clues as to their injuries or condition.

Unresponsive means that the casualty does not respond to voice or pain. But be aware that casualties do recover from this state.

While waiting for the ambulance, it is useful to record the state of impaired awareness and to note any changes in the casualty's condition – improvements as well as any deterioration.

FAINTING

Fainting fits into this chapter on unconsciousness because fainting is best described as a temporary loss of consciousness resulting from a reduction in blood flow to the brain.

A faint is often precipitated by an emotional upset or a surprise, but is most commonly due to physical inactivity – standing or sitting still – particularly in a warm environment. The classic faint victim is the soldier on parade. Blood is returned to the heart through the squeezing effect of muscles on the veins. When the muscles in the leg are not being exercised, blood flow to the heart is reduced, which reduces the amount of blood, and oxygen, being fed to the brain. The body's solution to this is to fall down and by doing so increase blood flow to the brain. A faint is, therefore, only the body's way of coping with a problem.

SIGNS AND SYMPTOMS

As the blood supply to the brain is restricted, the potential signs and symptoms of a faint may be present some time before the casualty actually faints.

■ *Pale skin*

■ *Slow pulse*

■ *Confusion and dizziness*

■ *Nausea and vomiting, leading to a brief loss of consciousness*

TREATMENT

STEP 1
Check Airway and Breathing.

STEP 2
Raise the legs to increase blood supply to the brain. If consciousness is not regained within one minute, turn the casualty into the recovery position and treat for unconsciousness.

STEP 3
Loosen tight clothing and ensure that the casualty has a good supply of air.

STEP 4
Do not let the casualty sit up too quickly. If you are unsure of the reason for the faint, advise the casualty to see their doctor.

If the casualty is simply feeling faint, lying them down with their legs raised should prevent a faint occurring.

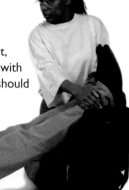

Dealing with Choking

CHOKING IS A FREQUENT PROBLEM
suffered by adults and is among the
most common causes of death in infants
and young children.

In a certain large fast-food chain in
America it is mandatory that the staff are
trained in choking procedures as it is an
almost daily event. Eating while driving
(not to be encouraged anyway because it
leads to a lack of concentration) also
increases the likelihood of choking on food.

Choking is defined as an object in the
throat blocking the airway, or inducing a
spasm of the air passages. This chapter
deals with the simple mechanisms which
can clear a blocked airway, and it examines
the differences between adults, children
and infants.

TREATMENT

There are three general procedures which
can be attempted to try to remove objects
blocking the airway. These, as shown on
the following pages, are adapted for use on
either conscious or unconscious casualties
and are used in different combinations on
adults, children and infants.

THE PROCEDURES

Back slaps
Abdominal thrusts
Chest thrusts

SIGNS AND SYMPTOMS OF CHOKING

You may be tempted to think that
anyone choking will be obvious.
However, it is not unknown for a
diner to collapse into their food
before anybody realises that they
are in trouble. If somebody is truly
choking they are unable to speak
and are generally unable to make
other sounds. Signs and symptoms
may include:

■ *Red-coloured face as they
struggle for air*

■ *As the oxygen supply to the
brain reduces, the casualty will
eventually become paler and
the lips may turn a blue-grey
colour (known as cyanosis)*

■ *Casualty may clutch at their
throat or at clothing around
their throat*

■ *Pulse rate will increase*

■ *Unconsciousness will result*

■ *Breathing will stop and,
eventually, so may the
circulation.*

CHOKING ADULT

CONSCIOUS ADULT

STEP 1

Encourage the casualty to cough.

STEP 2

If coughing is ineffective, lean the casualty forward and hit them firmly between the shoulder blades, using the flat of your hand. Give up to five sharp slaps.

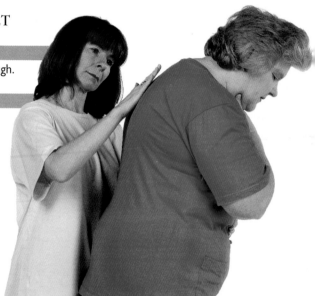

STEP 3

If the object still hasn't come up and the casualty is still choking, try the abdominal thrust, again up to five times. Put your hands around the casualty's body underneath their rib cage. Link your hands and pull inwards and upwards. This has the effect of forcing the diaphragm upwards and pushing the air out of the air passages. Hopefully this will take the foreign body with it. (Be warned the object can come out with some force.)

STEP 4

Continue alternating the back slaps and abdominal thrusts until the object is cleared. However, if the object does not come up, ensure that an ambulance has been called.

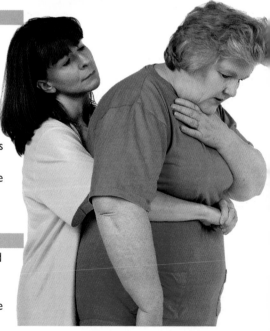

UNCONSCIOUS ADULT

If you know the casualty has choked and that they are now unconscious, you can adapt the back slaps and abdominal thrusts.

STEP 1

Open the casualty's airway using the jaw lift and head tilt (see page21).

STEP 2

Assess their breathing – the relaxation of the muscles due to unconsciousness may have released the obstruction allowing the casualty to breathe again. If they are breathing, or they start to breathe again at any point during these steps, turn them into the recovery position (see pages 23–25). Call an ambulance and monitor the casualty's condition. If they are not breathing, attempt artificial ventilations (see page 40).

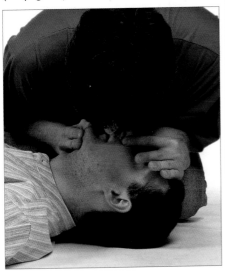

STEP 3

If you are unable to ventilate the casualty, turn them onto their side and give up to five sharp blows between their shoulder blades, using the flat of your hand. Check the mouth and, using a finger, hook out any loose objects.

STEP 4

If back slaps fail, you need to sit either astride or alongside the casualty. Place the heel of your hand below their ribcage and place your other hand on top, interlocking the fingers. Press sharply up towards the diaphragm up to five times.

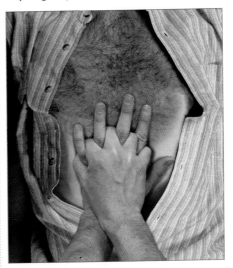

STEP 5

If the casualty is still not breathing, ensure that an ambulance has been called. Try mouth-to-mouth and, if the chest does not rise, repeat steps 3 and 4 until either the ambulance arrives or the casualty starts to breathe.

CHOKING CHILD

CONSCIOUS CHILD

Generally, a child is considered to be up to age seven. However, you need to use your judgement – for example, use adult mechanisms for a large seven-year-old and maybe child procedures for a small ten-year-old.

STEP 1

Bend the child over your lap, with the head lower than their chest (gravity can help). Hit them on the back up to five times, using the flat of your hand. Check their mouth and remove any obvious obstruction.

STEP 2

If this does not work, try up to five chest thrusts. Stand or kneel behind the child and place your fist against their lower breastbone. Grasp it with your other hand and pull inwards at a rate of one thrust every three seconds. Check their mouth and remove any obvious obstruction.

STEP 3

If step 2 does not work, try abdominal thrusts. Make a fist and place it against the child's central upper abdomen. Grasp this fist with your other hand and push inwards and upwards towards the diaphragm up to five times. Check their mouth and remove any obvious obstruction.

STEP 4

If the obstruction has still not cleared and the child is still choking, call an ambulance. Repeat steps 1–3 until help arrives or until the obstruction is cleared.

UNCONSCIOUS CHILD

If you know that the child was choking before they went unconscious, you can adapt the back slaps, chests thrusts and abdominal thrusts for use on a child who is lying down.

STEP 1

Open the child's airway using the head tilt and jaw lift (see page 21) and assess for breathing. If they are breathing, or they start breathing again during any of this process, turn them into the recovery position (see pages 23–25). Call an ambulance and monitor the child's condition.

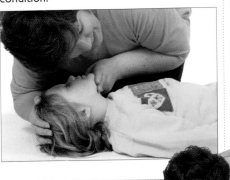

STEP 2

If they are not breathing attempt artificial ventilations (see page 45).

STEP 3

If you cannot ventilate the child, turn them onto their side and give up to five back slaps, using the flat of your hand. Then repeat step 1.

STEP 4

If you still cannot ventilate the casualty, turn them face upwards on the floor and give up to five sharp downward thrusts onto the lower half of the chest bone, pressing at a rate of once every three seconds. Compress the chest to a third of its depth. Then repeat step 1.

STEP 5

If you are still unable get air into the casualty, place the heel of your hand between the child's navel and breastbone and give up to five abdominal thrusts (inwards and upwards towards the diaphragm). Repeat step 1.

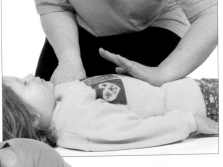

STEP 6

Call for an ambulance.

STEP 7

Repeat steps 3–5 until help arrives.

CHOKING INFANT

An infant is generally considered to be up to one year of age.

STEP 1

Lay a conscious infant face down on your forearm, ensuring that the neck and head are supported. Give up to five sharp slaps on the casualty's back.

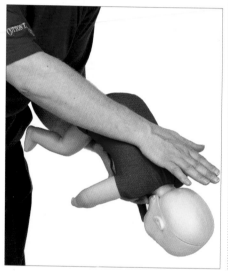

⚠️ **DO NOT FEEL** down the throat of an infant or a child. It can aggravate a potentially fatal condition known as *epiglottitis*.

⚠️ **DO NOT USE ABDOMINAL** thrusts on an infant. If the baby becomes unconscious, carry out the resuscitation sequence shown on pages 46–47.

STEP 2

Check the casualty's mouth, and remove any obvious obstructions with one finger.

STEP 3

If this has not cleared the obstruction and the child is still choking, turn the casualty over so that they are lying face down along your arm (or lay them on your lap), with the head supported. Using two fingers, compress the chest to a third of the depth giving up to five sharp thrusts. Then repeat step 2.

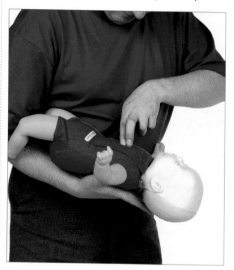

STEP 4

If the obstruction has still not cleared, repeat stages 1–3 a further three times. Then, taking the baby with you, call for an ambulance.

Cardio-pulmonary Resuscitation

THE BODY NEEDS OXYGEN TO SURVIVE. Oxygen is drawn into the body through the process of breathing and is carried around the body in the blood to the tissues and organs. Blood is circulated by the pumping action of the heart through the circulatory system, which consists of arteries, veins and capillaries (see *pages 53–54 for more detail*).

Without oxygen, the vital organs – particularly the brain – will not be able to function, and eventually death will result. This chapter looks further at the concept of ABC and considers what to do in the absence of breathing (respiratory arrest) and circulation (cardiac arrest).

This process of assessing and dealing with the non-breathing casualty and the casualty whose heart has stopped is known as resuscitation.

The resuscitation sequence is fundamentally the same, regardless of whether you are dealing with an adult, infant or child. However, there are obviously slight differences because of the variations in size and physiology.

I will look at each of these stages in detail on the following pages, but first we need to consider the concept of the Chain of Survival.

RESUSCITATION SEQUENCE

The resuscitation sequence builds on the checks and actions introduced in the chapter on dealing with the unconscious casualty (*pages 17-30*) and moves on to consider the actions necessary for dealing with non-breathing casualties and casualties without a heartbeat.

- ■ *Check for danger*

- ■ *Assess the casualty to see if they are conscious*

- ■ *Airway – open the airway*

- ■ *Breathing – check the breathing and, if necessary, breathe for the casualty*

- ■ *Circulation – check for circulation and, if necessary, circulate blood for the casualty*

- ■ *Call for help at the earliest appropriate time*

THE CHAIN OF SURVIVAL

To give a casualty suffering from cardiac failure the best chance of survival, it is essential that all four of the following steps can be undertaken as early as possible.

EARLY CALL FOR HELP

EARLY CARDIO-PULMONARY RESUSCITATION

EARLY DEFIBRILLATION

EARLY ADVANCED CARDIAC CARE

EARLY PHONE CALL It is essential with respiratory or cardiac arrest to get professional medical help as soon as possible. The panel immediately to the right gives the optimum time of calling for an ambulance during the resuscitation sequence.

CARDIO-PULMONARY RESUSCITATION CPR is the process of providing a casualty with oxygen (artificial ventilation) and circulating the oxygen in the blood around the body (chest compression). CPR in itself will not generally restart the heart or restore breathing. Its role is more that of a heart-lung (cardio-pulmonary) machine providing oxygen to keep the vital organs alive and to prevent brain death.

EARLY DEFIBRILLATION A defibrillator delivers an electric shock across the heart, which is often effective in restarting the heart's own rhythm. While defibrillators will not save every victim of cardiac arrest, they are a very effective tool. It has been estimated that for every minute that passes between cardiac arrest and defibrillation, the chances of survival decline by 10%.

EARLY ADVANCED CARDIAC CARE Hospitals today often have specialised cardiac care units, and research has provided great developments in the care of victims recovering from cardiac arrest.

WHEN TO CALL AN AMBULANCE

As I have said, calling an ambulance is a key component to resuscitation.

- If you have a helper send them for the ambulance as early as possible.

- If you are alone and the casualty is a child, or a victim of drowning or injury, carry out the resuscitation sequence for one minute (either ten breaths if they have a pulse, or one minute of CPR if the circulation is not present).

- If you are alone and the casualty is an adult and there are no signs of injury or drowning, call for an ambulance as soon as you realise that the casualty is not breathing. On your return to the casualty, continue with the resuscitation sequence.

RESUSCITATION IN ADULTS

The first steps of this process are exactly the same as for any unconscious casualty, but before you do anything, remember to check for danger.

STEP 1
Assess whether or not the casualty is conscious.

STEP 2
Open the casualty's airway by lifting the jaw and tilting the head.

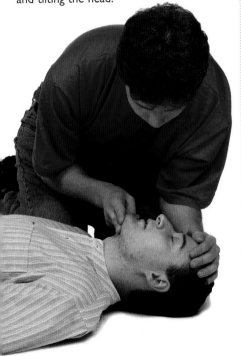

STEP 3
Listen, look and feel for breathing.

If the casualty is not breathing you need to ventilate them (see *page 40*) by using the oxygen that remains in the air you breathe out. There is more than enough oxygen in your expired air to keep the casualty alive.

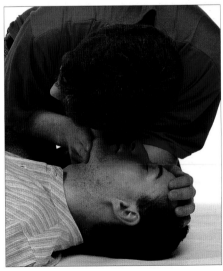

PERFORMING ARTIFICIAL VENTILATIONS

STEP 1
Remove any obvious obstructions from the mouth. With the head extended and the jaw lifted, pinch the casualty's nose shut.

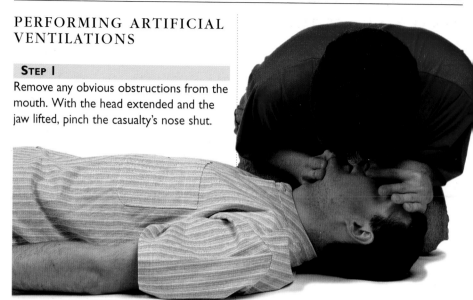

STEP 2
Place your lips around the casualty's mouth and breathe out (into the casualty's airway), taking approximately two seconds to inflate their lungs.

STEP 3
Take your mouth away from the casualty's mouth and watch the chest drop.

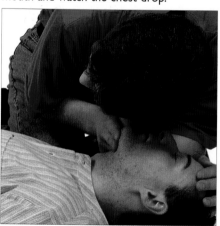

STEP 4
Repeat the procedure, giving the casualty two breaths in total.

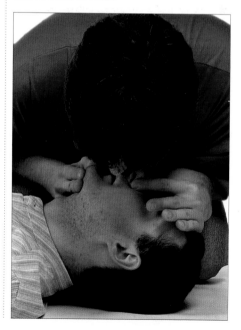

WHAT TO DO IF THE CHEST DOES NOT RISE

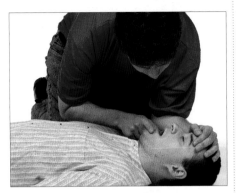

- Recheck the mouth and remove any obvious obstructions.
- Check that the head is tilted and the jaw lifted.
- Check that the nose is fully sealed.
- Ensure that you have sealed all the way around the casualty's mouth.
- Try up to five times to inflate the lungs.

If this does not work, and you do not suspect that the casualty has choked on something, go on to check the circulation, taking the pulse at the carotid artery, and continue with the resuscitation sequence (see page 37).

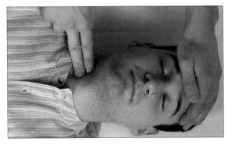

If you do suspect choking, try the procedures for an unconscious choking adult (see page 33).

GIVING ARTIFICIAL VENTILATIONS TO A CASUALTY IN THE CAR

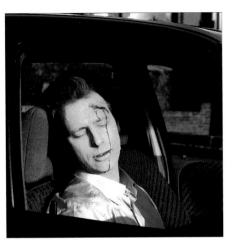

Mouth-to-mouth can be given to a casualty in a car. Gently tilt the head back and lift the jaw to open the airway. Give ventilations as described on page 40. If you suspect that the casualty is vomiting, they should either be leaned forward or removed from the car to ensure vomit can drain out.

⚠ IF THE CASUALTY starts to breathe, maintain an open airway by tilting the head back (see page 21).

⚠ IF AT ANY POINT you believe that circulation has ceased, you need to remove the casualty carefully from the car and start chest compression (see page 42).

CHEST COMPRESSIONS

Check the casualty's circulation by taking the pulse in the neck for up to ten seconds while looking for other signs of a circulation, such as movement or breathing.

If you are sure that the pulse is present, continue the ventilations, giving ten breaths, before rechecking the pulse. Continue with a cycle of ten ventilations and then a pulse check.

If you believe that circulation has stopped, you need to give the casualty chest compressions.

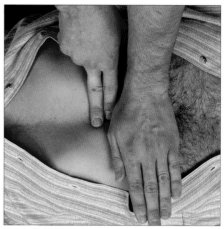

To find the correct position on the sternum, use two fingers on your free hand to find the depression where the ribcage gives way to the upper abdomen. Place the heel of your compressing hand immediately above.

STEP 1
Kneel next to the casualty.

STEP 2
Place the heel of your hand on the lower half of the sternum.

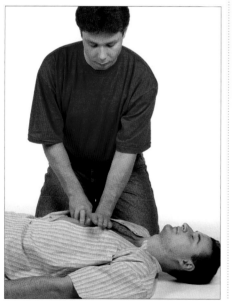

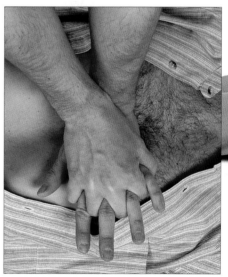

STEP 3
Place your other hand on top and interlock the fingers, pulling them off the chest to reduce the risk of damage to the ribs.

STEP 4

Lock your elbows straight and push down, compressing the chest 4–5 cm at a rate of 100 a minute (slightly faster than one per second).

STEP 5

Compress the chest 15 times.

STEP 6

Give two breaths.

STEP 7

Repeat the cycle of 15 compressions to two artificial ventilations until either the ambulance arrives or you notice signs of the casualty's recovery.

RECAP

Check for danger.

Assess the casualty's condition.

Open the casualty's AIRWAY.

Check the casualty's BREATHING.

If breathing, turn the casulaty into the recovery position.

If not breathing, give the casualty two artificial ventilations, inflating for approximately two seconds.

Check the casualty's CIRCULATION for up to ten seconds.

If circulation is present, continue with ventilations, rechecking the circulation every ten breaths.

If circulation is absent, alternate 15 chest compressions, at a rate of 100 a minute and a depth of 4-5 cms, with two ventilations.

Ensure that an ambulance has been called at the earliest appropriate opportunity.

RESUSCITATION IN CHILDREN

Having checked for danger and assessed the casualty's condition, you need to open the airway in the same way that you would for an adult – two fingers to lift the chin and a hand on the forehead to tilt the head backwards.

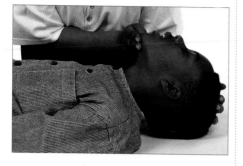

⚠ A CHILD IS CONSIDERED to be up to age seven. However, you need to use your judgement – for example, use adult mechanisms for a large seven-year-old and possibly child procedures for a small ten-year-old. The general rule is that if you have to shift your position while moving from artificial ventilations to chest compressions, you should try the adult CPR process on the larger child.

CHECK BREATHING

STEP 1

Check the breathing for up to ten seconds.

STEP 2

If the casualty is breathing, place them in the recovery position (see pages 23–25).

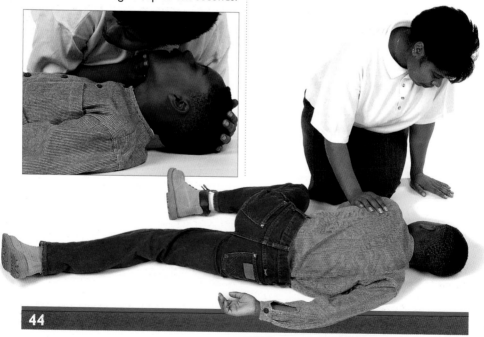

STEP 3

Check the mouth for any obvious obstructions. If they are not breathing, give five breaths of artificial ventilation by pinching the nose and sealing your mouth around their mouth and breathing out into their airway.

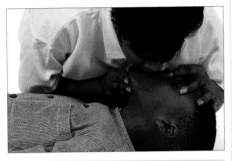

STEP 4

Move on to check the circulation.

CHECK CIRCULATION

STEP 1

Check the pulse in the carotid artery for up to ten seconds, while looking for other signs of recovery.

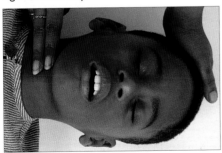

STEP 2

If you are sure that you can feel a pulse and you are alone, continue ventilation for one further minute before calling for an ambulance. On returning from the phone, continue ventilations, checking for circulation every minute.

STEP 3

If the circulation is absent, move on to chest compression.

CHEST COMPRESSIONS

STEP 1

Place the heel of your hand on the lower half of the breast bone and compress to a third of the depth of the chest at a rate of 100 a minute.

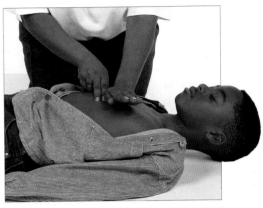

STEP 2

Give five compressions to every one ventilation.

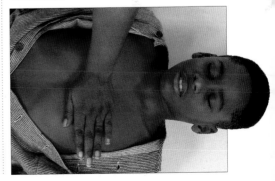

RESUSCITATION IN INFANTS

Having checked for danger, you need to assess whether the casualty is conscious by gently shaking the infant, and then open the airway.

CHECK BREATHING

STEP 1

Infants have very delicate windpipes and fragile necks. Open the airway gently, using one finger to lift the jaw, and carefully move the head back.

STEP 2

Check for breathing for up to 10 seconds.

STEP 3

If the infant is breathing, hold them in your arms on their side to help maintain an open airway.

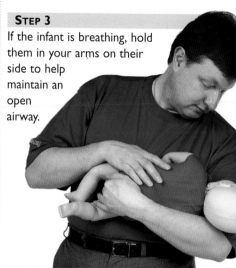

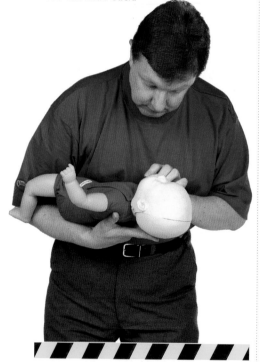

⚠️ AN INFANT IS CONSIDERED to be up to about one year old.

STEP 4

Remove any obstructions from the mouth. If the infant is not breathing, give artificial ventilations. Place your mouth over the casualty's mouth and nose. Gently breathe into the mouth and nose, watching for the chest to rise.

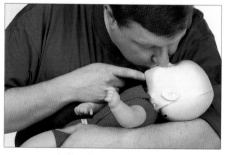

STEP 5

Give five breaths before moving on to check the circulation.

CHECK CIRCULATION

As babies' necks are so fragile, the pulse should be checked in the brachial artery in the arm (see page 54).

STEP 1
Check the pulse for up to ten seconds, looking for signs of circulation.

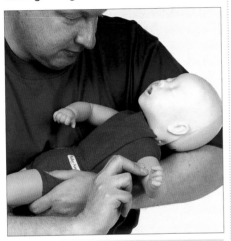

STEP 2
If you can feel a pulse of over 60 beats a minute, continue ventilations for one minute if you are alone before going to call for an ambulance.

STEP 3
On returning from the telephone, continue ventilation, rechecking the circulation every minute.

STEP 4
If you believe that there may not be a circulation or the pulse rate is less than 60 beats a minute, you need to combine chest compressions with your ventilations for one minute before going for the phone.

CHEST COMPRESSIONS

STEP 1
Place two fingers on the lower half of the breast bone.

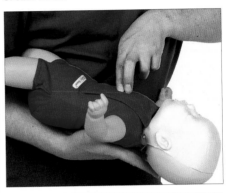

STEP 2
Compress the chest to a third of its depth at a rate of 100 a minute.

STEP 3
Give five compressions to every one ventilation.

CALLING AN AMBULANCE

If possible, take the infant with you to the telephone, and continue resuscitation.

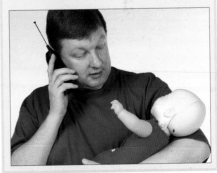

RESUSCITATION IN SPECIAL CIRCUMSTANCES

MOUTH-TO-NOSE RESUSCITATION

There may be circumstances when mouth-to-mouth resuscitation is difficult – corrosive liquids around the mouth, for example, or a badly broken jaw. Mouth-to-nose resuscitation is an acceptable alternative in these situations.

STEP 1
Tilt the casualty's head back in the same way you would for mouth-to-mouth resuscitation (see page 40).

STEP 2
Close the casualty's jaw and place your thumb over their mouth.

STEP 3
Seal your mouth over the casualty's nose and breathe out into the casualty's airway until the chest rises.

STEP 4
Remove your mouth to let the air escape.

MOUTH-TO-STOMA RESUSCITATION

In some rare cases an individual may, as a result of some illness or accident, be breathing through a hole in their neck known as a *stoma*.

In these situations you need to seal your mouth around the stoma and breathe into the casualty, watching for their chest to rise.

If the chest does not rise and the air escapes through the mouth and/or nose, it may be that the casualty is what is known as a 'partial breather'. In this situation you need to seal off the mouth and nose with your hand before breathing into the casualty.

BARRIER METHODS

Some first aiders may wish to use face shields or masks when giving mouth-to-mouth resuscitation. While many of these devices are very simple to use, it is important that you have practised with them first. Your local Red Cross branch will often be able to give you an opportunity to do this.

It is important that you carry your mask or shield with you everywhere – but if you do not have one to hand, this should not prevent you from attempting resuscitation.

Dealing with Shock

IN THE FOLLOWING CHAPTER, I SHALL be discussing wounds and bleeding, but before I move onto that fundamental subject for the first aider, it is important to mention shock.

The reason why bleeding is so dangerous is that it is one of the major causes of physical shock (also known as *hypovolaemic* shock). This is a condition resulting from a loss of circulating body fluid – the blood – and should not be confused with the emotional shock that might occur, say, when you have won the lottery or received bad news (although the external signs are often very similar).

In external bleeding this loss of circulating body fluid is obvious – the blood is generally very visible! With internal bleeding the loss of vital fluids may not be so obvious, and for this reason it is important that you learn to recognise the condition. Shock kills, so it is vital that you can recognise the signs and symptoms, which are detailed in the panel at the top of page 50.

OTHER CAUSES OF SHOCK
Shock is not only related to bleeding. Other causes include burns, fractures, heart problems, vomiting and diarrhoea. These are discussed in more detail in their relative chapters, but be aware that throughout *First Aid for Motorists*, you will be directed to look at this chapter whenever the subject of shock arises.

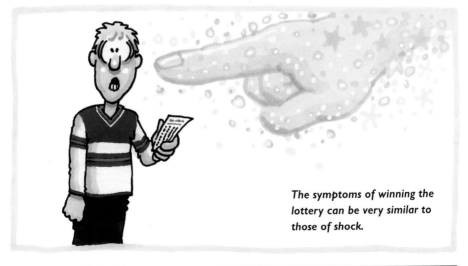

The symptoms of winning the lottery can be very similar to those of shock.

SIGNS AND SYMPTOMS OF SHOCK

- *Pale, cold and clammy skin*

- *Fast and weak pulse*

- *Fast and shallow breathing*

- *Dizziness and weakness*

- *Confusion*

- *Unconsciousness*

- *Breathing and heartbeat stopping*

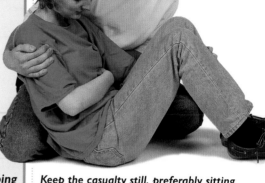

Keep the casualty still, preferably sitting down against a support, or lying down if they feel giddy.

A severe loss of body fluid leads to a drop in blood pressure. Eventually the blood's circulation around the body deteriorates and the remaining blood flow is directed to the vital organs (brain, heart, lungs, liver and kidneys). Blood is therefore directed away from the outer areas of the body so that the casualty appears paler than they were previously, and their skin feels cold and clammy.

As blood flow diminishes so does the amount of oxygen reaching the brain, so the casualty may appear to be confused, weak and dizzy, and may eventually deteriorate into unconsciousness. To compensate for this lack of oxygen, the heart and breathing rates both speed up. They also become gradually weaker and, if not treated, may eventually cease.

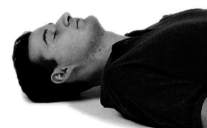

Keeping the casualty's head low may prevent the loss of consciousness.

SHOCK CAN OCCUR some time after an accident, particularly with internal bleeding. If a casualty with a history of injury displays the symptoms of shock coupled with any of the symptoms of internal bleeding, they should be advised to seek medical attention with some urgency.

TREATMENT OF SHOCK

The treatment of shock is best remembered by using the following mnemonic:

WARMTH

(Warmth, Air, Rest, Mental rest, Treatment, Help)

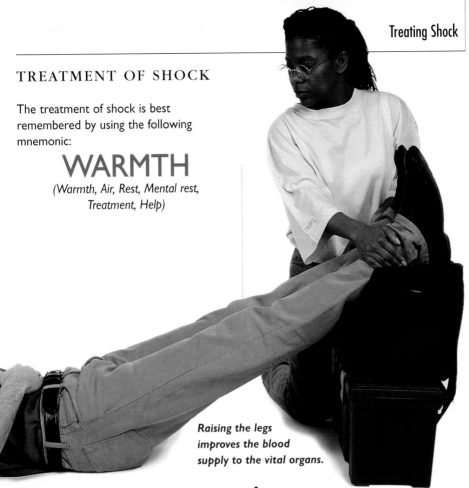

Raising the legs improves the blood supply to the vital organs.

WARMTH

In dealing with shock, it is important that the casualty is not allowed to get cold. Where possible they should be protected from the elements – if the car is safe, the best place for a casualty to stay after a car accident is in the vehicle itself; they are, after all, designed to protect us from the elements. If the casualty is on the ground, try to get something underneath them as well as over them; this is where your blanket in the boot is essential – alternatively use coats, jackets, jumpers, or whatever else is to hand or may be borrowed from other bystanders.

AIR

Maintain a careful eye on the casualty's airway and be prepared to turn them into the recovery position if necessary (see pages 23–25), or even to resuscitate if they stop breathing. Loosen tight clothing and try to clear back bystanders to allow maximum air to the casualty.

REST

Keep the casualty still, preferably sitting or lying down. If they are giddy, lay them down, legs up in the air, to ensure that the maximum of blood – and therefore maximum of oxygen – is sent to the brain.

MENTAL REST

Reassure the casualty… but be realistic. It is no good telling an injured person that everything is going to be fine if it is obvious that there is something seriously wrong; they will lose all faith in your ability as a first aider. Let them know that everything that can be done is being done, and that help has been called for. If they have other worries (such as who will be picking up their child from school, or what has happened to their dog who was also in the vehicle), try to solve these problems for them. I once treated a motorcyclist who was far more concerned about the state of his new motorcycle than he was about his injured leg. As it turned out, the bike was much better off than he was.

TREATMENT

Treat the cause of the shock and aim to prevent fluid loss.

An injured casualty may suffer the effects of shock at any time, so even when they are lying in the recovery position, protect them from the cold with coats or blankets. Do not apply a hot-water bottle or other source of direct heat.

HELP

Ensure that appropriate medical help is on the way. Generally this will be the ambulance but it may be that you have to refer someone to the Accident and Emergency Department some days after the original accident.

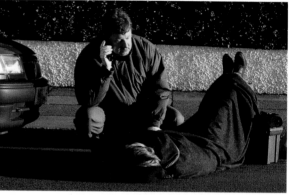

If the casualty is lying on cold ground, ensure there is a blanket underneath them as well as wrapped over the top. Reassure them that help has been called for.

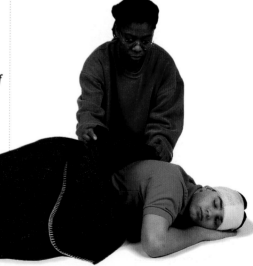

Dealing with Bleeding

MOST OF US HAVE CUT OURSELVES at some point in our lives; from paper cuts to grazed knees, we have all lost blood from our circulatory system. Generally this type of injury is little more than an annoyance, easily dealt with by adhesive plasters. But a large blood loss is a life-threatening occurrence, and it is this situation that I cover in this chapter.

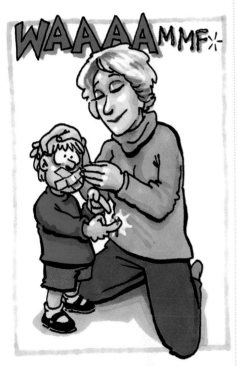

Most domestic incidences of bleeding can be treated with adhesive plaster and a little Tender Loving Care...

THE NATURE OF BLEEDING

Blood is carried around the body in three different types of vessel:

- arteries
- veins
- capillaries

ARTERIES have thick, elastic muscular walls which contract. It is this 'pumping' action that pushes blood out from the heart under pressure. Arterial blood is full of oxygen, which has been collected from the lungs, and the main function of arteries is to take this oxygen-rich blood to the organs and body tissues. Because the blood is under pressure and is so full of oxygen, an arterial bleed is characterised by bright red blood pumping from an injury. An arterial bleed is very serious as blood is quickly lost to the system.

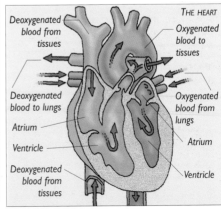

THE HEART

Deoxygenated blood from tissues

Oxygenated blood to tissues

Deoxygenated blood to lungs

Oxygenated blood from lungs

Atrium

Atrium

Ventricle

Ventricle

Deoxygenated blood from tissues

BSM

VEINS have thin walls and return blood from the organs and tissues to the heart. They do not have muscles of their own and rely on the actions of the muscles around them to squeeze the blood through the system. To ensure the blood moves in one direction around the body, veins have a series of one-way valves. When these valves deteriorate blood pools up in the veins making them swell. This weakens the vein wall resulting in a condition known as varicose veins.

While blood loss from a bleeding vein (a venous bleed) does not tend to be as quick as an arterial bleed, it still has the potential to be a serious, possibly fatal, injury. A venous bleed will appear to flow from an injury and, as it has little or no oxygen, it will appear to be a dark red.

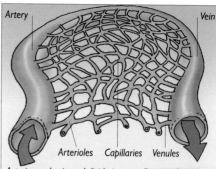

Arteries and veins subdivide into smaller vessels and then into thin-walled capillaries where material passes from the blood to the cells of the body tissue.

CAPILLARIES are very thin-walled vessels. Blood is forced through them under extreme pressure, which causes the food and oxygen stored in the blood to be pushed out into the body tissues and organs (see *above*).

CHECKING THE PULSE

The key reasons for checking the pulse are to determine whether:

- **the heart has stopped**
- **blood is flowing**
- **the casualty's circulation is satisfactory after applying bandages**
- **the casualty is suffering from shock.**

A pulse can be felt wherever an artery runs close to the surface of the skin and is caused by the pressure wave as blood passes through the circulatory system (*see also page 28*). As arteries contract with each heartbeat, the pulse can be used to determine how well the heart is functioning.

WHERE AND HOW TO CHECK

When checking for cardiac arrest, there are two places that the pulse should be read:

- **the carotid pulse in the neck**
- **the brachial pulse in the arm (particularly with infants).**

The most common place for taking the pulse for recording purposes is at the radial artery in the wrist. There is also a good pulse in the ankle that can be used to check for impaired circulation. Always use your fingers, not your thumb. The thumb has its own pulse which you might read by mistake. Take the pulse for one minute (or, if pressed, for 30 seconds and multiply the result by 2).

TYPES OF INJURY

Bleeding can be both external and internal. External bleeding involves a break to the skin surface. This break, known as a wound, can take many different forms.

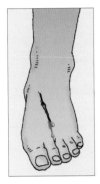

INCISED WOUND

Clean, deep cuts – such as those caused by paper and knives – are known as incisions. There may be underlying damage to tendons and other tissues and considerable blood loss.

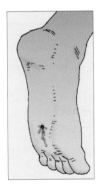

PUNCTURE WOUND

These wounds are deep injuries caused by a long needle-like object. Although they do not bleed a great deal, puncture wounds carry the risk of infection if dirt is carried deep into the tissue.

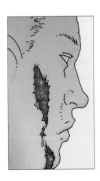

LACERATION

For motorists involved in car accidents, the most likely injury is a laceration – a jagged wound which tends to bleed a lot and which carries a high risk of infection.

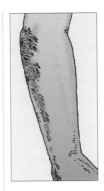

ABRASION

Abrasions (grazes) are commonplace injuries involving damage to the top layer of the skin. They rarely bleed a lot, but are often dirty because of the debris embedded within them.

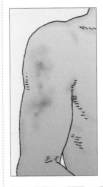

INTERNAL BLEEDING

This is often caused by a blunt blow. It is common in traffic accidents where sudden deceleration can throw motorists forward. Bruising is a supeficial form of internal bleeding.

THE CLASSIC EXAMPLE of internal bleeding is where a motorist, stopped suddenly, has been thrown against the seatbelt. This violent deceleration causes internal bleeding. Serious internal bleeding is no less dangerous than external bleeding – in fact, as there is little that can be done by the first aider to control internal bleeding, it has the potential to be life-threatening. If it is suspected, the first aider should call for medical aid as soon as possible.

EXTERNAL BLEEDING

External bleeding can be frightening. While intelligent care should always be taken over any bleeding, it may be a cliché to say but it really does often look worse than it is. Imagine pouring half a litre of milk over the floor; it will probably spread out across half of the kitchen. Now consider the panic that you would feel if that same surface area was covered by blood. And yet this amount is only as much as many people give freely at a blood donor session with few, if any, ill effects.

Serious shock in an adult usually develops only after a litre or more of blood is lost from the body, and even this can be treated effectively with good first aid and early hospital care.

PROTECT AGAINST INFECTION. Sources of infection may be contained in all body fluids. You and the casualty may be at risk if you have an open cut or sores, especially on your hands. Carry a supply of disposable gloves with you (*see page 10*) – at the scene of an accident you are unlikely to be able to wash your hands before treating anyone, and the gloves will protect the casualty, as well as you. In any event, ensure that you wash your hands thoroughly as soon afterwards as possible.

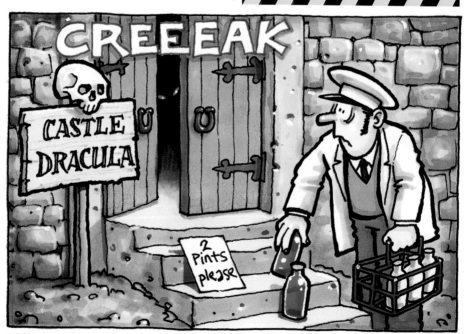

Half a litre of blood is only as much as many people give at a blood donation centre.

THE TREATMENT

The four main principles of the treatment of external bleeding are:

1. Look
2. Apply pressure
3. Elevate
4. Treat for shock (see pages 50–52)

STEP 1

Look at the wound to check its extent. Look for secondary areas of bleeding, as the pain from one wound might mask the pain from another. Check that the wound has nothing embedded in it – known as a foreign body (see pages 58–59).

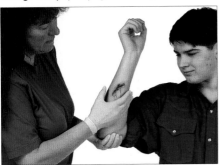

STEP 2

Apply pressure to the wound. If the casualty is able to press on the wound themselves, encourage them to do so. If not, apply pressure yourself, initially with your fingers and, if you have something to hand, eventually a sterile dressing or a piece of clean cloth.

Applying pressure to the wound enables the blood to clot and therefore stems the blood flow from the cut. Once applied, a sterile dressing (or whatever you have to hand) should ideally be held in place with a firm bandage or improvised bandage, such as a scarf or a tie.

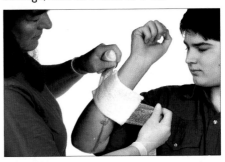

STEP 3

If the injury is on an arm or leg, elevate the wound above the level of the heart. As it is harder for blood to pump uphill, elevating the injured part reduces the blood flow to the wound and consequently also reduces the fluid loss from the body.

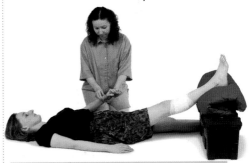

STEP 4

All the time that you are dealing with the wound, treat the casualty for shock (see pages 50–52) and remember to tell them what you are doing in order to reassure and keep them calm.

More detailed information on some specific wound sites may be found on pages 60–61, but generally these principles apply to any wound, whatever its size and wherever it is on the body.

BSM

WHAT IF SOMETHING IS STUCK IN THE WOUND?

Those of you with an eye for gory detail will remember the television reconstructions of the sportsman with the javelin through his neck and the lorry driver with a steel pole through his stomach. Both of these casualties lived without any long-term problems thanks to the general principles of dealing with a foreign body in a wound (and some heavy duty cutting equipment courtesy of the fire brigade). Hopefully you will never have to deal with anything of that magnitude, but the general principles are the same for a piece of glass as they are for a spear.

⚠️ DO NOT REMOVE THE OBJECT. If it went in at an angle you may cause more damage by pulling it out. You may leave splinters in the wound. The object may be pressing against a vein or an artery, reducing blood loss. You may have mistaken a broken bone for a foreign body.

⚠️ IF THE CASUALTY IS IMPALED on something which cannot be moved, support them to stop them from pulling on the impaled object and causing further damage. Where possible treat them as described above, and ensure that the emergency services are aware of the need for cutting equipment.

THE TREATMENT

STEP I

Apply pressure around the edges of the wound using your hands without pressing on the foreign object.

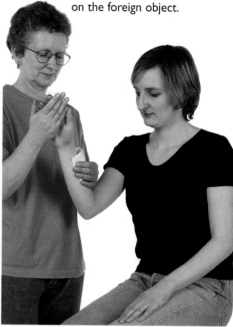

STEP 2

Replace this pressure with a sterile dressing. Using clean pads, build a bridge either side of the wound to protect it.

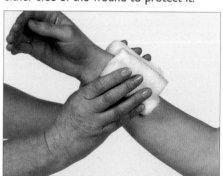

STEP 3
Bandage firmly in place.

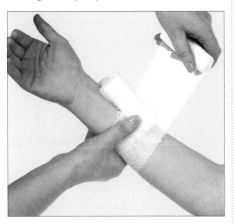

STEP 4
Elevate injured limbs if possible.

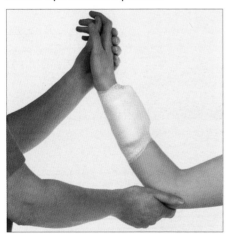

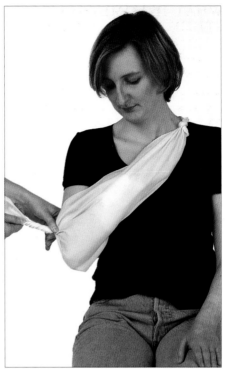

An arm wound with a foreign body in it can be kept elevated after bandaging by using an elevation sling (see page 76). Take care not to move the embedded object when putting the sling in place.

STEP 5
Prevent longer objects from moving by supporting them with your hands or by packing a coat around the base of the object.

STEP 6
Treat for shock (see pages 50–52).

BLEEDING FROM SPECIAL SITES

NOSE BLEED

First ensure that the casualty hasn't broken their nose (if they have, applying the following procedure is likely to get the first aider flattened!). If they haven't broken their nose, lean the casualty forward and encourage them to spit blood out into a handkerchief or some other receptacle. This will stop them from swallowing blood which is a sure-fire way to cause vomiting.

Do not pinch the nose if you suspect that the casualty may have broken their nose.

Next pinch the nose just below the hard bit towards the top (about one-third down the length of the nose) and apply firm pressure for ten minutes – it takes this time for a clot to form. If the bleeding hasn't stopped after ten minutes, apply pressure for two further periods of ten minutes. If it still hasn't stopped, either take or send the casualty to hospital.

Once the bleeding has stopped advise the casualty not to scratch, pick or blow their nose, not to drink hot drinks and not to exert themselves, because all of these can dislodge the clot and cause the bleeding to start again.

The situations described on these two pages may appear minor, but the casualty should be monitored for shock and treated if necessary, just as you would for more serious bleeding conditions. A conscious casualty should lie down with their head and shoulders raised. If they become unconscious, place them in the recovery position (*see pages 23-25*).

BLEEDING FROM THE EAR

If the blood from the ear is thin and watery because the blood is mixing with the fluid that cushions the brain, there may be some damage to the skull, and possibly the brain. This is a very serious injury. Call the emergency services as soon as possible. Keep the casualty still and gently rest the head, injured ear down, with a clean pad held over the ear for the blood to drain into. Do not tie this pad in place. Keep a check on the casualty's ABC and be prepared to resuscitate if necessary.

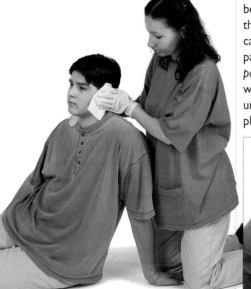

If the blood is bright red and is accompanied by earache, deafness, a sudden change in pressure or an explosion, this may indicate a burst eardrum. Again, keep the injured ear downwards, hold a clean pad in place and seek medical attention.

WOUNDS TO THE SCALP

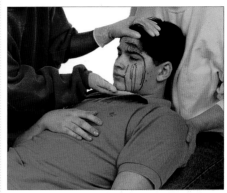

A scalp wound can appear worse than it is, because there is a rich supply of blood to the area. But the casualty should be carefully examined in case the wound is part of a more serious head injury (see page 69). Apply pressure to the wound with a sterile pad to bring the bleeding under control. Next, secure a fresh pad in place with a bandage.

TREATMENT OF INTERNAL BLEEDING

As was stated on page 55, this is potentially a very serious condition. While the blood may not be spilled onto the floor, it is still lost to the circulatory system and the casualty is very likely to go into shock.

WHAT TO LOOK FOR WITH INTERNAL BLEEDING

- *The history of the accident*

- *Signs and symptoms of shock*

- *Bruising*

- *Boarding – this most commonly occurs where there is bleeding into the stomach area; the quality of blood combined with the tissues swelling results in a rigidity to the tissues*

- *Swelling*

If you observe any combination of these signs and symptoms you should suspect internal bleeding. Treat the casualty for shock (see *pages 50–52*) and seek urgent medical attention.

Less serious internal bleeding (i.e. small bruises) can be treated with a cold compress to relieve pain and reduce swelling. However, the possibility of further internal bleeding or underlying injury should not be ruled out – particularly if the casualty has a history of a blunt injury such as hitting their head on a window after an accident or being hit in the stomach by a reversing car.

Your aims are to get the casualty to a hospital urgently and, while waiting for the ambulance, prevent shock (see pages 50–52). Raise and support the legs, take the pulse at the wrist, and keep the casualty warm (but never apply direct heat, such as a hot-water bottle).

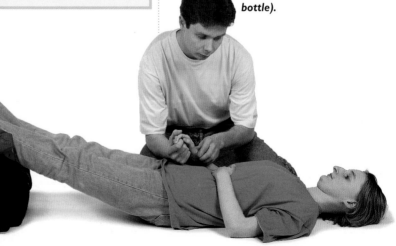

Dealing with Fractures

MANY OF US WILL HAVE SUFFERED either a broken bone or known someone who has. Fractures (the correct word for broken bones) are very common, generally painful but rarely life threatening. However, poor handling of fractures can lead to problems, and some fractures bring special complications with them. This chapter is intended to help you identify potential fractures. It will show you how to treat them in a way that reduces the risk of further damage to the casualty, and how to deal with the complications brought about by fractures to specific body sites.

TYPES OF FRACTURES

Having ascertained that fracture is just another word for break, we can identify two main types:

CLOSED FRACTURE Here the bone has broken and has not pierced the skin. These are often difficult to diagnose and will rely on an x-ray to determine whether or not the bone is definitely broken.

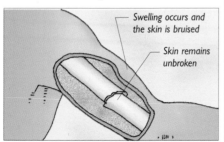

Swelling occurs and the skin is bruised

Skin remains unbroken

OPEN FRACTURE In this case the bone has either pushed through the skin or is associated with an open wound. The greatest risk with open fractures is infection.

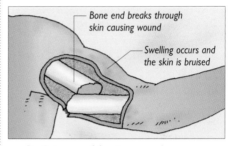

Bone end breaks through skin causing wound

Swelling occurs and the skin is bruised

Both types of fracture can be complicated because the injury has caused further damage to underlying organs or blood vessels.

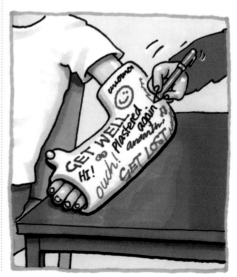

THE SKELETON

The human skeleton has a number of functions. In terms of first aid, the main ones to interest us are:

- protection for important organs and blood vessels
- a base for muscles, ligaments and tendons, which combined enable us to move (the skeletal muscular system).

There are some 206 bones in the body, but those most commonly broken are the 'long' bones in the arms and the legs.

SKULL
Damage to the skull can cause damage to the brain.

SPINE
If broken, the spine can cause damage to the spinal cord and the spinal circulation.

RIBS
There are 12 pairs of ribs, attached to the spine at the back and curving round to the front. Of these, 10 pairs are attached to the sternum at the front. Many of the vital organs lie beneath the ribs. An impact can cause the ribs to break and to move inwards, causing damage to the lungs, heart, liver and kidneys, and other internal bleeding.

UPPER ARM AND LEG
Sharp ends of broken bone can pierce the brachial (upper arm) and femoral (upper leg) arteries.

PELVIS
The pelvis protects the urinary system and a serious fracture can burst the bladder, leading to potential infection.

STERNUM
The sternum (breastbone) is joined to the ribs by cartilage to make the ribcage flexible for breathing. A broken sternum may press directly into the heart. However, it takes a considerable impact to cause these types of injury. They were often seen in pre-seatbelt days if the driver impacted with the steering wheel.

These potential complications are considered later in this chapter.

RECOGNISING FRACTURES

While it is possible to give a general guide to the recognition of fractures, no two people are identical in their responses. In one case a girl who had fallen badly from her bike refused treatment until she had finished the race she was participating in. It was only after she had completed the race and sought medical advice that it was realised that she had broken her pelvis and would require six weeks immobilisation. She shouldn't even have been able to walk let alone ride.

If in any doubt, therefore, the first general rule has to be to assume that there are fractures and treat the casualty as such. Be particularly aware of potential fractures if the accident involved a sharp impact to the point of injury, a fall, sudden acceleration/deceleration or a sudden twist. More detailed signs and symptoms of fractures can be remembered through the use of the mnemonic:

PADS CUTS
(Pain, Deformity, Swelling, Crepitus, Unnatural movement, Tenderness, Shock)

PAIN This accompanies most, but not all, fractures and is caused by the broken bone ends pushing onto nerve endings.

DEFORMITY An injured part may appear deformed particularly when compared to the uninjured side.

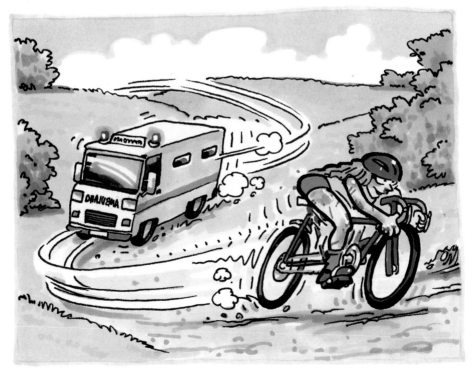

SWELLING An increase in blood to the tissues surrounding the injured part to help fight off infection cause swelling.

CREPITUS The sound of two broken bone ends rubbing together – if good first aid is being carried out this is not a sound you should hear.

UNNATURAL MOVEMENT The fracture, especially of limbs, means that an arm or leg may not move in their accustomed directions.

TENDERNESS This accompanies most fractures and is often felt only when the injured part is gently touched.

SHOCK The signs and symptoms of shock often accompany major fractures.

There may be reddening or bruising over the site of the fracture, but often this takes some time to appear and may not readily be a sign you can see at the accident.

If your casualty is displaying any combination of the above symptoms and/or there is evidence at the accident site to suggest a fracture may be likely, it is

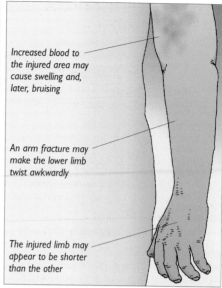

Increased blood to the injured area may cause swelling and, later, bruising

An arm fracture may make the lower limb twist awkwardly

The injured limb may appear to be shorter than the other

A bending, twisting or shortening of the limb may be apparent. Bruising and swelling may develop at the fracture site after the injury.

best to assume that a fracture is present.

Another potential sign of a fracture is a lack of feeling, or a pins and needles sensation, below the fracture site. This may indicate nerve damage or a reduction in circulation caused by the bone pushing on either the nerves or the blood vessels.

The treatment for injuries displaying these symptoms is the same as for any fracture. However – and only if the first aider is properly trained – the application of traction may alleviate the problem.

The first priority is to keep the casualty still, and support the fracture.

GENERAL PRINCIPLES OF THE TREATMENT OF FRACTURES

The general rule for treating all fractures is to keep the casualty still. This reduces pain and the likelihood of further injury. This is a three-step process.

⚠ DO NOT MOVE the fracture unnecessarily, and be prepared for the casualty to tell you that they are quite all right by themselves, which leaves you free to keep them warm and to get help.

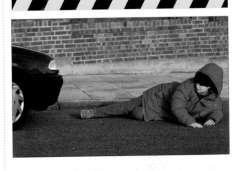

STEP 1

The casualty will often have moved the injured part into a position that is most comfortable for them and will almost certainly be keeping still. However, there are always exceptions to the rule and, if necessary, you should advise the casualty to keep still. If need be, help the casualty into a comfortable position.

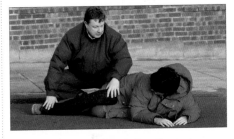

STEP 2

Once the casualty is still, you can help steady and support the fracture using your hands. By helping the casualty keep the injured part still, you enable them to relax. The very act of relaxing the muscles reduces the pull on the broken bones and often alleviates pain.

STEP 3

If you have to transport the casualty yourself, or if it is going to be a while until help arrives, you can immobilise the fracture further with bandages or by improvising with coats, blankets, etc. The key points to remember with any bandaging – improvised or using bandages from your kit – are:

■ not to tie the bandage too tightly
■ to pad around the site of the fracture.

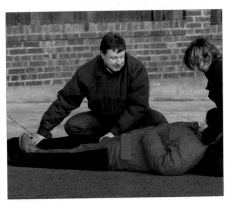

TREATMENT OF OPEN FRACTURES

While keeping the injury still is an important part of the treatment of open fractures, the risk of infection is also an important consideration – and it requires action. In the first instance the wound should be protected by either a sterile dressing or a dressing improvised from a piece of clean, dry and non-fluffy material. If the bleeding is profuse, or if you are going to have to wait some time for further help, this dressing should be held in place using the same principles you would apply if there was a foreign object in the wound (see *pages 58–59*).

STEP 1

Place the dressing over the wound and build up padding alongside the bone.

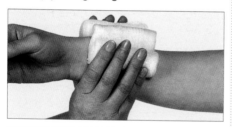

STEP 2

Tie both the padding and the dressing in place using firm pressure.

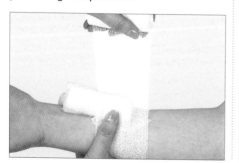

STEP 3

Remember that the tissues around fractures swell and you may need to loosen the bandage if the circulation becomes impaired below the site of the fracture.

CHECKING FOR CIRCULATION IMPAIRMENT

With any bandaging you run the risk of reducing the circulation of blood to body tissues below the bandage's position. In part this can be avoided by not tying bandages too tightly and by avoiding deliberate tourniquets altogether. But wounds tend to swell leading to a once satisfactory bandage becoming too tight. There are three ways to check whether a bandage is cutting off circulation:

1. Skin below the site of the bandage becomes white/grey/blue or feels cold to the touch.

2. Casualty complains of pins and needles or lack of circulation if the pulse in the limb slows or stops.

3. Colour does not return quickly to the skin after it is gently pinched or to the nail if it is compressed.

If you notice any of the signs or symptoms, gently loosen, but do not remove, the bandage until the blood flow returns.

FRACTURES OF THE SKULL AND FACE

A skull fracture is a very serious injury and is often associated with some form of injury to the brain. Concussion and compression may both accompany skull fractures (see *panel on page 70*).

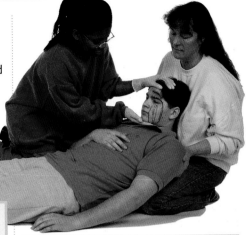

POTENTIAL SYMPTOMS OF A SKULL FRACTURE

- *Bruising to the eye socket*

- *Straw-coloured fluid coming from one or both ears or the nose*

- *A deterioration in the level of consciousness of the casualty*

If any of these symptoms are present, assume a skull fracture with underlying brain injury.

STEP 1
Keep the casualty still while they are conscious.

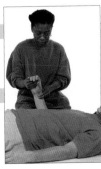

STEP 2
Keep a check on their ABC.

STEP 3
Be prepared to resuscitate or turn into recovery position if necessary.

STEP 4
Call for medical aid as soon as possible.

STEP 5
If there is fluid coming from the ear, place this ear downwards and cover it with a sterile pad. But do not plug the pad into the ear.

If there are fractures to the bones of the face and jaw, the airway is your overwhelming priority.

- Ensure that any blood in the mouth is allowed to dribble out – encourage the casualty to spit into a bandage or handkerchief.
- Gently remove any teeth or bits of broken bone from the mouth and give the casualty a pad to hold against the injured part for additional support and comfort.
- A cold compress may help reduce the pain but the general treatment is to get the casualty to hospital.
- Do not pinch a broken nose to control bleeding.

CONCUSSION AND COMPRESSION

CONCUSSION is a shaking of the brain caused by sudden movement of the head. It is a common condition in car accidents as the forward-and-backward movement of a car stopping suddenly moves the brain forward inside the skull. The casualty is likely to display a number of the following characteristics:

- **Pale skin**
- **Dizziness, nausea or blurred vision**
- **Headache**
- **Brief or partial loss of consciousness**

The casualty will recover when the disturbance caused by the shaking stops. However, because concussion often accompanies violent head movement, you should always suspect the possibility of a skull fracture or a more serious, longer-term brain injury, such as compression. So it is important that even seemingly recovered concussion casualties should be advised to seek medical treatment.

TREATMENT FOR CONCUSSION

1. Place in recovery position, if necessary, and monitor ABC.
2. Call an ambulance if the casualty does not recover after three minutes or if there are signs of skull fracture or compression.

3. Encourage the casualty to remain still while recovering to reduce dizziness and nausea.
4. Be aware of the increased likelihood of neck injuries.

COMPRESSION is a very serious injury that occurs when pressure is exerted on the brain, perhaps from a piece of bone, or bleeding or swelling of the injured brain. It may develop immediately after a head injury or stroke, or some hours or even days later. Potential signs and symptoms include:

- **Deterioration in the level of consciousness**
- **Flushed and dry skin**
- **Slurred speech and confusion**
- **Partial or total loss of movement, often down one side of the body**
- **Unequal pupils**
- **Noisy breathing which becomes slow**
- **Slow, strong pulse**

If some or all of these symptoms are present, suspect compression.

TREATMENT FOR COMPRESSION

1. If unconscious, place the casualty in the recovery position and monitor ABC. If conscious, lay the casualty down with their head and shoulders slightly raised, maintaining a close check on the ABC.
2. Call an ambulance.

FRACTURES OF THE SPINE

Unfortunately spinal injuries are common in car accidents, either because of the sharp fore-and-aft movement caused by sudden deceleration or by a direct impact onto the spine.

Most injuries occur around the neck area as the head is thrown violently forward on impact and then backward again. A properly adjusted car head-rest can reduce the risk of neck injuries by preventing the head from being thrown all the way back.

With spinal injuries, the greatest danger is the risk of nerve damage. The spinal cord containing the spinal nerve runs down through the centre of the vertebrae and fractures of the vertebrae can sever or pinch these nerves, leading to partial or full paralysis.

Although not all spinal fractures result in immediate damage to the spinal cord, the risk is greatly increased if bones are broken, so any suspected fracture of the spine should be treated with extreme care.

Conversely not all spinal-cord injury is caused by fractured vertebrae. Displaced vertebrae or swelling due to blood loss can apply pressure to the spinal cord, leading to nerve damage.

Suspect a fractured spine or potential nerve damage if the history of the accident involves:

- rapid deceleration
- a fall from a height
- a sharp blow directly to the back
- injury to the face or skull (this often results from the head being thrown back in a fore-and-aft movement).

SIGNS AND SYMPTOMS

SPINAL FRACTURE

- *A possible dent or step in the spine which may indicate a displaced vertebrae*
- *Bruising or swelling over the spinal column*
- *Complaint of pain in the back*
- *Tenderness over the area of the fracture*

SPINAL CORD DAMAGE

- *Loss of movement below the site of the fracture*
- *Pins and needles in the extremities or throughout the body*
- *A feeling of 'strangeness'; 'feeling like jelly' etc.*
- *Numbness*

If any of these symptoms are present – or if the accident history indicates a potential fracture – assume that a fracture is present.

The treatment for injuries to the spine is relatively simple: **KEEP THE CASUALTY STILL**. While the casualty's ABC will always come first, the general rule for dealing with fractures or spinal-cord damage is to keep the casualty in the position that you found them in, taking particular care to immobilise the head.

If you have been trained to do so, you can move the head into the neutral position before immobilisation.

CONSCIOUS CASUALTIES

If the casualty is still in their car seat, leave them there.

STEP 1
Tell them to keep still.

STEP 2
Try to prevent people moving around in the car as this will move your casualty.

STEP 3
Ensure that an ambulance has been called.

STEP 4
Hold the casualty's head still.

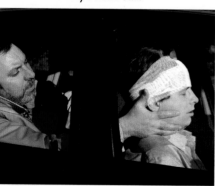

STEP 5
If it appears that there will be a long wait for the ambulance, and the injury is to the neck area, ask a bystander to improvise a neck collar using, for example, a jumper or a newspaper.

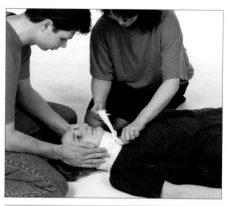

STEP 6
Do not remove your support from the head even once the collar has been applied.

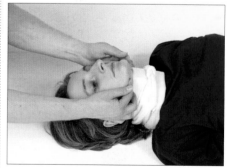

If the casualty is conscious and out of the car, gently get them to sit or lie down. Support their head as before, and apply a collar if it is appropriate.

UNCONSCIOUS CASUALTIES

The casualty's airway is always your first priority. They *may* have a broken spine, which *may* lead to nerve damage. But if you do not protect their airway they will die.

STEP 1
Carry out your ABC checks, taking care to tilt the head gently.

STEP 2
If the casualty is lying in such a way that their head is extended, and they are on their side, which will allow fluid to drain safely from the mouth, leave them there.

STEP 3
Hold the head as described in step 4 for conscious casualties, and ensure that their airway is monitored.

STEP 4
If the casualty's head is not extended or they are not lying on their side, you need to move them into the recovery position. Ideally this manoeuvre should be carried out with the assistance of a bystander (see *page 74*). If you are alone, be prepared to roll the casualty into the recovery position by yourself as detailed on pages 23–25.

NON-BREATHING CASUALTIES

Follow the resuscitation procedure detailed on pages 39–47. If you have to roll the casualty onto their back to resuscitate them, keep the head, trunk and toes in a straight line. If present, bystanders can help – but do not waste time looking for help – the casualty needs air urgently.

WHIPLASH
A common injury after sudden-impact car accidents, whiplash – best described as a 'neck sprain' – is an injury to the soft tissue of the neck that may need long-term physiotherapy and the use of a neck collar.

It is very difficult to distinguish whiplash from spinal-cord damage and neck fractures since the symptoms and potential accident histories are very similar. In fact, because spinal injuries and whiplash are caused in similar ways, they may both be present, and the pain of the whiplash injury may be masking other, more serious, problems.

For this reason whiplash should be treated in the same way as other spinal injuries until more serious damage is ruled out by professional medical staff.

SPINAL INJURY
RECOVERY POSITION

STEP 1
Support the casualty's head as described
above on page 73. Be comfortable, you may
have to do this until the ambulance arrives.

STEP 2
The bystander should put the arm nearest
them gently underneath the casualty's body,
ensuring that the fingers are flat and the
elbow straight.

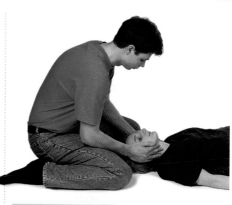

STEP 4
The casualty's furthest leg should be
bent upwards and the bystander's
arm placed on the thigh just
above the knee.

STEP 3
They should then bring the furthest arm
across the body supporting it at the face.

STEP 5
Working under orders from the first aider
at the head, the casualty should be turned
over, ensuring that the head, trunk and
toes stay in line.

STEP 6
Once in position, continue to support the
neck while the bystander makes the patient
stable, either by supporting the body
themselves, or by placing coats or a rolled
up blanket, etc, around the casualty.

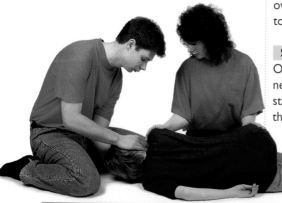

FRACTURES OF THE ARM AND WRIST

SLINGS

The long bones in the arm are among the most commonly broken. Generally, victims of broken arm bones can be transported to hospital by car, but the arm should be immobilised to prevent pain or any further damage while moving. This can be done either with an improvised sling made from clothing or by using a triangular bandage to form an arm sling.

STEP 1

Gently place the bandage under the casualty's arm, placing the point on the underneath of the injured elbow.

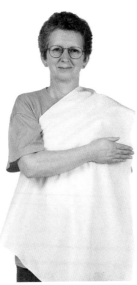

STEP 2

Pass the top end of the bandage around the back of the casualty's neck, leaving a short end to tie by the collar bone on the injured side.

STEP 3

Carefully bring up the bottom end of the bandage, ensuring that it fully supports the injured arm, and tie it into place with a reef knot (or failing that a bow). Tighten at the elbow.

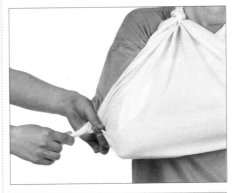

STEP 4

For additional support you can tie another triangular bandage folded into three (a broad fold) around the arm, avoiding the site of the fracture, to stop the arm from moving.

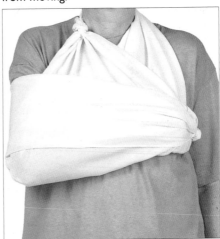

BSM

ELEVATION SLING

This alternative to the arm sling shown on page 75 is used for fractures to the hand or collar bone. It can also be used to elevate the arm in the treatment of burns and bleeding.

STEP 1
Place the injured arm with the fingers by the collar bone on the uninjured side.

STEP 2
Place the triangular bandage with the point resting at the elbow on the injured side.

STEP 3
Tuck the bandage underneath the hand and down underneath the injured arm.

STEP 4
Take the end under the shoulder blade and tie at the collar bone.

STEP 5
Fasten the spare material at the elbow with a pin, or twist it and tuck it away.

STEP 6
Extra support can be provided by placing a triangular bandage folded into three (a broadfold) around the arm and body.

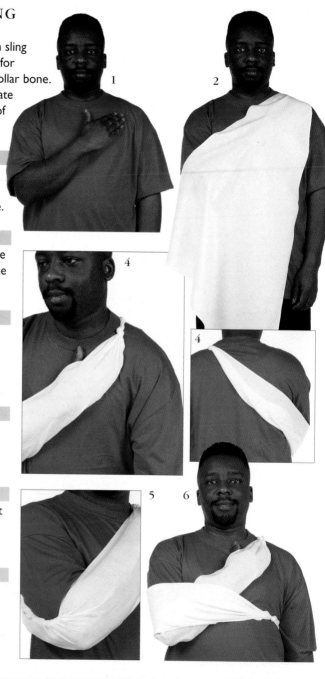

76

IMMOBILISING THE LEG

As fractures of the legs will generally require transportation by ambulance, the general treatment is simple. Hold the injured part still and treat the casualty for shock. Support the leg above and below the site of the fracture, if possible, placing padding around the broken leg to further help to reduce movement of the injured limb. If you have been trained in the use of traction, you may apply this gently to the leg to help to reduce pain and circulatory damage.

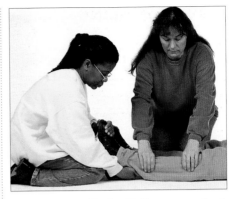

Hold the injured limb still. If you are trained to do so, gentle traction will ease the pain.

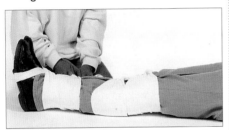

Strapping the injured leg to the uninjured leg, with padding between, will help reduce movement and further damage.

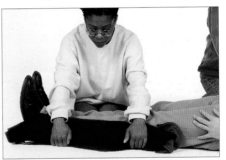

Reduce movement of the injured part by placing rolled-up blankets beside it.

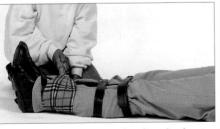

If you do not have a supply of medical bandages with which to strap the legs, scarves and belts can be used to improvise.

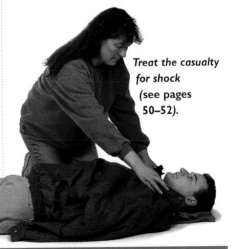

Treat the casualty for shock (see pages 50–52).

FRACTURES OF THE PELVIS

Although the pelvis is a large bone and generally difficult to break, fractures of the pelvis, or hip bone, are common in car crashes and when pedestrians have been hit by a vehicle. Because the bone protects the urinary system, the biggest danger is that sharp bone ends may burst the bladder, creating the possibility of infection. And because the pelvis is difficult to break, it implies a heavy-impact accident if it is broken, which in turn means the likelihood of internal bleeding should be suspected.

SIGNS AND SYMPTOMS

- *Bruising and swelling over the hip area*

- *A feeling of wanting to go to the toilet*

- *Blood-stained urine*

- *The sensation that they are 'falling apart' (the pelvis is a like a girdle and a fracture means that the girdle may not be holding itself together)*

- *Legs rotated outwards as the support at the 'girdle' gives way*

⚠️ A PELVIS BROKEN at the back is easy to mistake for a spinal injury. If in doubt, treat the casualty for a fractured spine.

TREATMENT FOR A FRACTURED PELVIS

STEP 1
Ask the casualty if raising their knees would make them feel more comfortable; this relieves the muscular pull on the pelvis. If they agree, gently bend and raise the knees, placing an improvised cushion (coat, blanket, etc.) underneath.

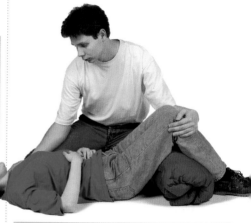

STEP 2
If the ambulance will be some time in arriving, the legs can be tied together gently at the ankles and knees, using triangular or improvised bandages and padding between the legs.

STEP 3
Treat the casualty for shock.

FRACTURES OF THE RIBCAGE

SIMPLE FRACTURES

Simple fractures are usually confined to one broken rib and with no underlying damage to the lungs or other internal organs. Characterised by bruising and tenderness over the fracture site, the best treatment for a simple fractured rib is to put the arm on the injured side into an arm sling and advise the casualty to seek medical aid.

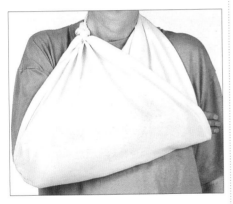

MULTIPLE RIB FRACTURES

Rib injuries involving more than one fracture (also called 'complicated rib fractures') often result in the casualty having difficulty in breathing because the chest wall is unable to move effectively. There may also be associated lung damage where one or more ribs has punctured one or both of the lungs.

Complicated rib fractures may include damage to the sternum and may lead to a condition known as 'flail chest'. In this condition the injured area moves in as the casualty breathes out and vice versa.

This is known as 'paradoxical breathing' and may lead to a lack of oxygen.

There may also be an open fracture of the chest wall where ribs have sprung out. Remember that the ribs extend around to the casualty's back and there may be injuries there as well as on the front.

The injures may be accompanied by a sucking wound to the chest. Here there is a direct passage between the outside and the lungs, often caused by a puncture injury from, in this instance, a rib.

SIGNS AND SYMPTOMS

- *Paradoxical breathing*

- *Swelling or indentation along the line of the ribs*

- *Open fractures*

- *Difficulty in breathing*

- *Pain on breathing*

- *Shock (there is likely to be some degree of internal bleeding)*

- *Bright red frothy blood coming from the mouth and/or nose (this is an indication of a punctured lung, as oxygenated blood is escaping from the respiratory system. There may or may not be an associated sucking wound to the chest)*

- *Sucking wound to the chest*

BSM

TREATMENT OF MULTIPLE RIB FRACTURES

STEP 1

If the casualty is conscious, lay them down, or they may find breathing easier in a half-sitting position.

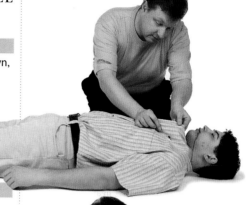

STEP 2

Lean the casualty towards their injured side. This allows any blood to drain into the injured lung leaving the good lung free to breathe.

STEP 3

Treat any sucking wounds (see *below*).

STEP 4

Treat any open fractures (see *page 68*).

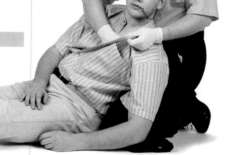

STEP 5

Place the arm on the injured side into an elevation sling (see *page 76*).

STEP 6

Treat the casualty for shock (see *pages 50–52*).

If the casualty becomes unconscious, monitor their ABC and place them into the recovery position with their uninjured side upwards.

SOFT-TISSUE INJURIES

Sprains and strains are best fitted into this chapter on fractures since they are often caused in the same way and are generally hard to distinguish from broken bones.

STRAINS are an overstretching of the muscle leading to a partial tear.

RUPTURES are complete tears in muscles.

SPRAINS are injuries to a ligament at or near a joint.

The symptoms will be similar to those of a fracture and will generally follow a sharp twisting or stretching movement.
   If both you and the casualty are confident that the injury is not fractured (and often the casualty has done this before and so will be the best judge), the best treatment is:

RICE

(Rest, Ice, Compression, Elevation)

STEP 1

Place the injured part at rest.

STEP 2

Apply a cold compress.

STEP 3

Apply a compressing roller bandage to help reduce pain.

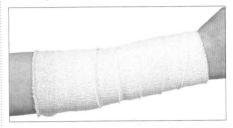

STEP 4

Elevate the injured part.

STEP 5

Seek medical aid.

If in doubt, treat the injury as a fracture.

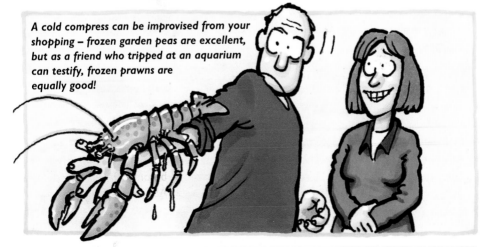

A cold compress can be improvised from your shopping – frozen garden peas are excellent, but as a friend who tripped at an aquarium can testify, frozen prawns are equally good!

DISLOCATIONS

WHAT IS A DISLOCATION?

A dislocation is the displacement of a bone or joint. The most commonly dislocated bones are those at the 'ball and socket' joints, most notably the shoulder.

One of the key dangers with dislocations is the risk of trapping nerves or blood vessels, which can lead to a long-term disability. However, effective first aid and early medical care can help reduce this risk.

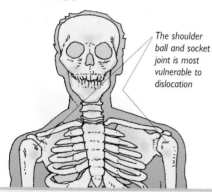

The shoulder ball and socket joint is most vulnerable to dislocation

SIGNS AND SYMPTOMS

■ *Sharp pain at the joint*

■ *Deformity at and around the joint (this may be noticed only when compared to the uninjured joint)*

■ *Potential pins and needles or numbness in the area below the dislocation, due to nerve damage or impaired circulation*

■ *Lack of, or reduced, movement at the joint*

TREATMENT

STEP 1

Help the casualty support the injured part in the most comfortable position. With a dislocated shoulder, the best way of providing this support is with an arm sling.

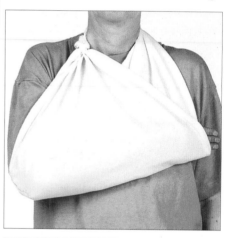

STEP 2

Ensure that the casualty receives prompt medical attention.

⚠️ DO NOT MAKE ANY ATTEMPT to move the dislocated bone back into its joint.

Dealing with Burns

WHILE I HAVE SAID THAT MOST CARS do not burst into flames, there is – since a burn can be caused in many ways – a risk of burn injuries to the car driver and other road users. In this chapter we look at the causes of burns, how to determine the severity of a burn injury and, of course, how to treat such injuries.

CAUSES OF BURNS

DRY HEAT	This is the most common type of burn and includes burns caused by hot objects, exhausts for example, or by flames, from a cigarette or lighter for instance.
WET HEAT	Also known as a 'scald', wet heat is generally taken to mean hot water or steam (from, say, a car's radiator). However, it can also include other hot liquids such as oil or fat.
FRICTION	When two objects rub together very quickly the friction generates heat, which can cause another kind of dry burn. Motorcyclists and pedal cyclists who don't wear appropriate protective clothing are among the most common victims of friction burns.
CHEMICAL	Acids and alkalis, both industrial and those in everyday use, can cause serious burns. Battery acid is caustic and can cause nasty burns if it comes into direct contact with the skin.
ELECTRICAL	These can be caused by the everyday low voltage currents found in the home or through arcing from the high voltage cables that you see scattered around the countryside. In rarer cases electrical burns can be caused by lightning strikes.
RADIATION	While this may sound drastic, most of us have suffered some degree of radiation burn at some point in our life – most commonly known as 'sunburn'. This complaint is very common to cyclists in the summer, particularly on the back of the neck, and can be associated with heat stroke, a potentially fatal condition which is described in more detail on page 96.

THE RISK FROM BURNS

As with any injury which loses fluid to the circulatory system there is a risk of **SHOCK**. In burns, fluid is lost in three main ways:

- *blistering*
- *swelling around the injury*
- *direct plasma loss through damaged tissue*

While the fluid loss may not be visible as liquid pooled around the casualty, it is, nevertheless, lost to the system. And so severe burns can, and often do, prove to be fatal.

The second risk from burns is through **INFECTION**. The damaged tissue provides little or no resistance to infection, and serious problems can set in early on in the treatment of a burns casualty which may not have an effect for some time after the initial injury.

ASSESSING THE SEVERITY OF A BURN

Most of us will have burnt ourselves at some point: sunburn, taking the joint out of the oven, falling down a grassy bank and ending up with friction burns. But few of us were probably in any real danger of suffering shock as a result, and there would have been little risk of a serious infection – so how do you determine when a burn is sufficiently serious to merit medical aid?

There are two main points to consider:

- *the depth of the burn*
- *the percentage of the body area which is burnt*

THE DEPTH OF THE BURN

Fans of television hospital series and crime fiction may be familiar with the old classification system of first-, second- and third-degree burns. But nowadays burns are classified into:

- *Superficial*
- *Partial thickness*
- *Full thickness*

SUPERFICIAL

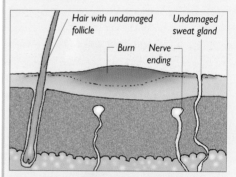

Hair with undamaged follicle — Undamaged sweat gland — Burn — Nerve ending

Burns of this type only involve the outer layer of the skin. While often extremely painful, they are not generally life-threatening unless a very large surface area of the body is covered (*see percentage area of the body burnt, page 86*).

The burnt area is very sore, usually red and possibly a little bit swollen. If good first aid treatment is applied and the area burnt is not extensive, further medical treatment is unlikely to be needed.

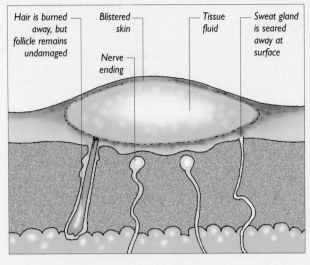

Hair is burned away, but follicle remains undamaged

Blistered skin

Nerve ending

Tissue fluid

Sweat gland is seared away at surface

PARTIAL THICKNESS

These burns include the top layers of skin and involve blistering. The risk of shock is high and any burn of this type needs medical attention to some degree. Partial thickness burns covering a substantial percentage of the body can kill. Partial thickness burns are characterised by red, raw looking skin, with blistering and pain.

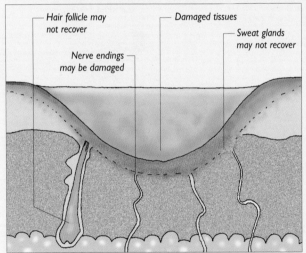

Hair follicle may not recover

Nerve endings may be damaged

Damaged tissues

Sweat glands may not recover

FULL THICKNESS

These burns involve damage to all the layers of skin. There is usually damage to nerve endings and possibly to other underlying tissues and organs. Characterised by charred tissue often surrounded by white waxy areas of dead skin (which sometimes doesn't hurt because of the nerve damage), full thickness burns will always need emergency medical attention. In the long term they frequently mean the casualty having to undergo plastic surgery.

PERCENTAGE AREA OF THE BODY BURNT

As a guide to whether urgent medical treatment is required in the case of a burn casualty, the 'rule of nines' can be applied. Dividing the body up into 9% sections (see below) makes it easier for a first aider and medical worker to determine the extent of a burn.

■ Any partial thickness burn of 1% or more needs medical attention. This need not be an emergency services call if adequate first aid treatment has been applied. If there are no other injuries, it may be sufficient to take the casualty to hospital (or a local health centre) yourself.

■ Any partial thickness burn of 9% or more needs urgent medical treatment, as the risk of shock is high. Call for an ambulance.

■ Any full thickness burn needs urgent medical attention and you should call for an ambulance as soon as you can.

If the casualty has other injuries, appears to be in a great deal of pain, is suffering from shock or you have other reasons to suspect that their condition is more serious, do not hesitate to call 999 whatever the extent or depth of the burn.

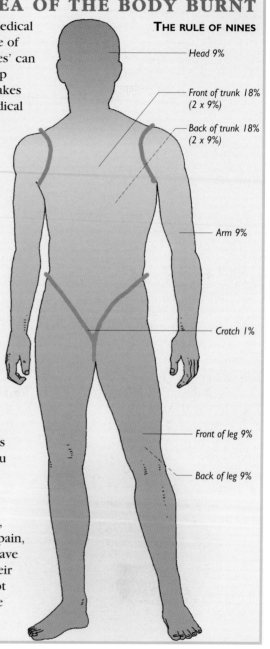

THE RULE OF NINES

Head 9%

Front of trunk 18% (2 x 9%)

Back of trunk 18% (2 x 9%)

Arm 9%

Crotch 1%

Front of leg 9%

Back of leg 9%

TREATMENT OF BURNS

In principle, the general treatment of all burns is very simple:

COOL & COVER

Below we look at the in-depth treatment for any burns. This is summarised on page 89.

STEP 1

The first priority at any accident is to protect yourself. This is particularly important with burns incidents. Ensure that the fire is out, that any electrical equipment is safely disconnected or that chemical spills are not going to affect you.

> ⚠ DO NOT OVER-COOL the casualty – restrict the cool liquid to the injured part where possible, as over-cooling could lead to hypothermia, particularly if the surrounding air temperature is low.

> ⚠ DO NOT APPLY WATER under pressure. If you are applying water from a shower, hose or even a gushing tap, ensure that the pressure is at a minimum – water hitting burnt skin at speed adds to both the pain and the damage.

STEP 2

Checking the casualty's ABC remains important, particularly if there are burns to the mouth and airway (see pages 20–28).

STEP 3

Douse the burnt area with cool liquid. Cooling the burn will reduce the pain, swelling and risk of scarring.

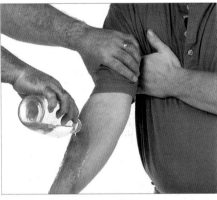

STEP 4

Treat the casualty for shock (see pages 50–52).

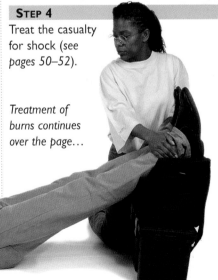

Treatment of burns continues over the page…

STEP 5
Make an assessment about whether or not an ambulance is needed and call for help. If in doubt call 999.

STEP 6
Keep cooling the injured part until the pain stops. Often ten minutes is sufficient, but if the casualty still complains of pain after this time, continue with the cooling treatment.

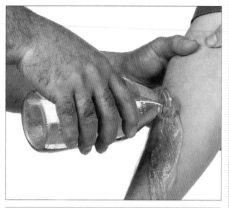

STEP 7
Remove rings, watches and other potentially constricting items – burns swell up and such objects could impair circulation. (Remember to return property or put the removed items in the casualty's pockets. You would not be the first first aider to walk away from an accident scene with a casualty's watch in your pocket.)

STEP 8
Once the pain has eased, cover the wound to prevent infection with a sterile bandage tied loosely over the burn. You can improvise with any clean, non-fluffy material, such as clean handkerchiefs or cotton pillowcases. Suitable bandages for burns can be seen on pages 92–93.

STEP 9
If possible, elevate the injured part to help to reduce swelling. Wait with the casualty until help arrives or, if the burn is less serious, accompany them to further medical attention.

⚠ DO NOT REMOVE burnt clothing sticking to the wound.

⚠ DO NOT PUT COTTON WOOL or other fluffy material onto a burn or it will stick to the injury.

⚠ DO NOT PUT ANY CREAMS or ointments onto a burn as this will need to be removed at the hospital.

⚠ DO NOT BURST BLISTERS as this may increase the risk of infection.

⚠ DO CONTINUE to treat for shock.

⚠ DO MAINTAIN a check on the casualty's airway, breathing and circulation.

⚠ DO CHECK bandages to ensure that they are not too tight.

BURNS TO THE NECK AND MOUTH

Beyond the risk of shock and infection, the greatest potential problem with burns to the neck and mouth is the risk of airway obstruction due to swelling.

If a casualty has burns in these areas the treatment is:

STEP 1
Check on the casualty's ABC and be prepared to resuscitate if necessary.

STEP 2
Call an ambulance.

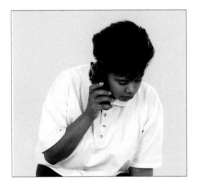

STEP 3
Get the casualty into a position that they feel comfortable breathing in (this will usually be sitting up).

STEP 4
Loosen any constriction around the neck.

STEP 5
Cool any burns continuously – do not attempt to cover.

STEP 6
Maintain a check on the casualty's ABC.

TREATMENT OF BURNS SUMMARY

1. Check for danger

2. Assess ABC (be prepared to resuscitate if necessary)

3. Cool the injured part

4. Make an appropriate decision about what help is required and call for an ambulance if necessary

5. Cover the injured part

6. Treat for shock throughout your treatment of the burn

7. Elevate the injured part if possible.

CHEMICAL AND ELECTRICAL BURNS

SPECIAL CONSIDERATIONS

While the general rules for the treatment of burns are the same regardless of the type of burn, there are some additional considerations that must be taken into account for chemical and electrical burns.

CHEMICAL BURNS

The key point when dealing with chemicals is not to contaminate yourself.

I have referred to HAZCHEM symbols on page 16, and the same rule applies here. If you are in any doubt about the nature of the chemical involved, get away from the casualty, get everyone else away and call for professional help.

If you feel that you can safely approach the casualty, there are some additional steps to add to the treatment:

- If necessary wear protective clothing.
- Ventilate enclosed areas because many chemicals affect respiration.
- When cooling down burns with water, ensure that the contaminated water runs away from both the casualty and yourself (as shown to the right).
- It may be necessary to flood the injured part for longer than ten minutes to ensure that the chemical is totally washed away.
- Inform the ambulance service that you are dealing with a chemical burn. Additional help may be needed from the fire service, and specific antidotes can be sent with the ambulance.

- If possible, remove contaminated clothes from the casualty as these will keep burning – but only do this if you can do it without contaminating yourself or harming the casualty any further.

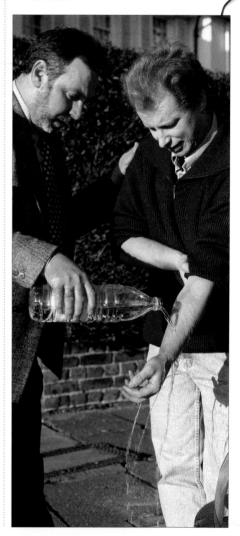

ELECTRICAL BURNS

The first point to remember is that because water is a good conductor of electricity, there is an obvious danger in using it with electrical burns, or if any electricity is present around the accident site. The points listed below are special considerations when dealing with electrocution cases:

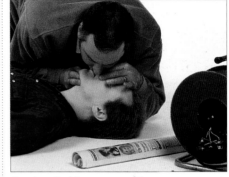

- Do not attempt to touch the casualty unless you are absolutely sure that they are no longer in contact with live equipment.
- If they are still attached to an electrical current, your best option is to turn off the electricity at the mains point.
- If you cannot access the mains you may be able to turn off electrical equipment at a wall socket.
- If you can't turn off the electricity, try to move the casualty away from the contact by using a non-conducting material, such as a broom handle (rubber gloves would also be useful). Insulate yourself from the ground by using rubber shoes, or standing on non-conductive objects that may be to hand, a pile of car manuals or a thick road atlas, for example.

An electrical burn may well cause respiratory or circulatory difficulties. An electrical discharge across the heart can cause cardiac arrest, so resuscitation may be necessary before treatment of the burn.

Electricity commands respect – if in doubt call in professional help.

METHODS OF COVERING BURNS

One of the best ways to cover a burn is to use clean triangular bandages. The bandage shown here can be used for the hand and adapted for use on the foot.

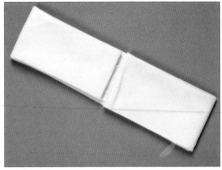
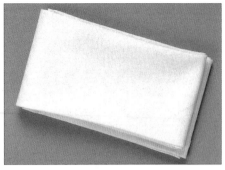

Place a sterile dressing or clean piece of material over the burn. Place a large pad on top of this to protect the area and absorb any plasma.

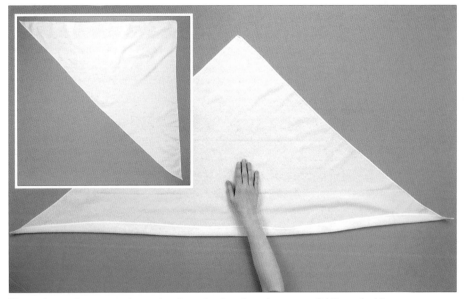

If you do not have a ready-made triangular bandage (see page 94 for suitable alternatives), cut a triangular shape from clean cloth (inset, above), approximately 1.4 metres along the base and 85 cm along the other two sides. As the long base of the bandage will be exposed after enclosing the hand, fold it over to make a hem which will keep it tidy. Place the casualty's hand on the bandage, as shown above.

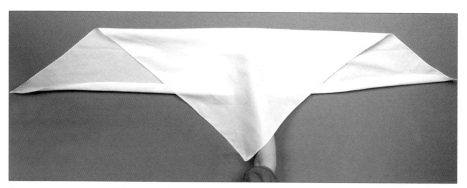

Bring the top point of the triangle down over the top of the injured part towards the casualty's wrist until the fold meets the point of the fingers (or toes).

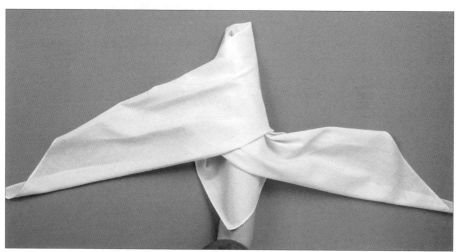

Cross the two ends of the bandage around the wrist and tie loosely.

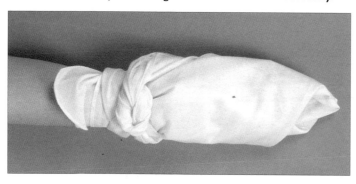

Pull the point of the bandage up over the knot and tuck it away.

USING A TRIANGULAR BANDAGE FOR ANY OTHER AREA

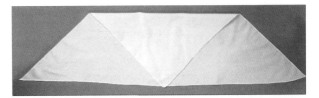

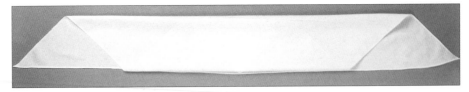

Folded over once (top) and then again into a broadfold (above), the triangular bandage can be used to hold a dressing and pad in place anywhere on the body, including extra support for arm slings. Or it can be folded once more (below) to be used as a bandage to control bleeding.

ALTERNATIVES TO BANDAGES

If you do not have sterile dressings available, cotton pillow cases and sheets are ideal substitutes – particularly for larger areas of burnt tissue.

A less obvious substitute is plastic film wrap such as you use in the kitchen. The film only sticks to itself and so won't stick to the burnt area. It provides a barrier to infection but allows medical staff to see the wound without having to take off bandages in the first instance. Tear off the first few wraps of the roll and loosely cover up the sterile dressing over the burn.

Another alternative for hand and foot injuries is to place the wounded part into an empty, clean sandwich bag (*right*).

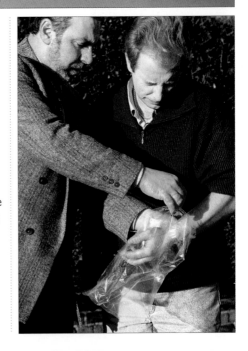

SUNBURN

Sunburn may seem the least dramatic of burn injuries, but there are two good reasons why it is included here. First, sunburn *can* be prevented. Second, it *is* a serious issue.

The very nature of first aid is in dealing with accidents – situations which cannot be prevented (although they can often be avoided) – and burns are invariably caused through accidents. Except for sunburn. Prevention is better than cure and it is relatively easy to avoid getting sunburn.

Prolonged exposure to the sun's ultra-violet rays can cause painful and potentially serious burns, and even heat-stroke (see *page 96*).

In the long term, sunburn can even lead to skin cancer.

There are three simple rules for prevention of sun-related problems, and they are:

SLIP, SLOP, SLAP

(Slip into a T-shirt – bare skin burns,
Slop on the appropriate sun cream
for your skin type,
Slap on a hat)

It is as well to remember that burning can happen even on cloudy days. Motorists' Arm is a common burn – driving with your arm resting on the window leaves a somewhat uneven tan...

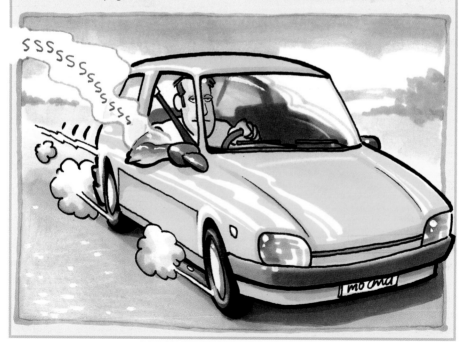

HEAT EXHAUSTION AND HEAT-STROKE

HEAT EXHAUSTION

Heat exhaustion is a condition resulting from the loss of fluid and salt, usually through excessive sweating. It is most common when a person has exerted themselves and not replaced fluid content – cyclists and joggers are frequent sufferers of heat exhaustion. The condition is very similar to shock in that fluid is being lost to the body. The signs and symptoms are similar too:

- **Pale, cold and clammy skin**
- **Fast and weak pulse**
- **Fast and shallow breathing**
- **Nausea, dizziness, disorientation**
- **Deterioration into unconsciousness**

TREATMENT
- Lay the casualty down in a cool place and raise their legs.
- If the casualty is conscious, give them sips of a weak salt solution (one teaspoon to one litre of water).
- Maintain a check on the casualty's consciousness level. If it deteriorates, place the casualty in the recovery position and call an ambulance.
- If the casualty's condition improves rapidly, advise them to see their own doctor.

HEAT-STROKE

Heat-stroke generally occurs when the brain's temperature regulator fails to work effectively. This tends to occur when the casualty has been in a very hot environment, or when they have a fever caused by a condition such as malaria.

The body becomes extremely hot very quickly, and this condition can be fatal. The signs and symptoms are very similar to those of a stroke (see page 110):

- **Hot, flushed and dry skin**
- **Slow, full and bounding pulse**
- **Possibly noisy breathing**
- **High body temperature**
- **Headache**
- **Disorientation**
- **Deterioration into unconsciousness**

TREATMENT
- Check ABC. If the casualty is unconscious turn into recovery position. Resuscitate if necessary. Call an ambulance.
- Move a conscious casualty to a cool environment. If this is impossible, or the casualty is unconscious, try to cool down the environment (use fans, open doors and keep crowds away).
- Remove outer clothes and wrap the casualty in a cold and wet sheet, and keep it wet.
- Continue the cooling process. If the body temperature drops, replace the wet sheet with a dry one.
- Continue to monitor the casualty.

First Aid and Specific Road Users

WHILE THIS BOOK IS AIMED AT THE motorist it is also important to consider other road users. Often enough the first person to come across an injured cyclist or pedestrian is a motorist.

This chapter identifies the common injuries faced by drivers and other road users, and advises the first aider on what they should be looking for.

DRIVER

INJURY	CAUSED BY	TREATMENT
Whiplash-strained muscles on the neck	Sudden deceleration	Keep the casualty still and treat as for fracture of the neck/spine (see pages 71–74)
Fractured neck/spine	Rapid deceleration and impact	Keep the casualty still, particularly the head. Apply an improvised neck collar if you suspect that the neck is broken (see page 27)
Bruising and possible internal injuries	Caused by the seatbelt digging into casualty after stopping suddenly. You may see 'pattern bruising' – bruising over the areas covered by the seatbelt	Treat the casualty for shock (see pages 50–52) and keep them as still as possible
Chest injuries	Impact on steering wheel (less common since the advent of seatbelt)	Treat fractures as described on pages 79–80. If the lung is punctured lean the casualty onto their injured side to allow the good lung to breath (see pages 79–80)
Head injuries	Hitting head on steering wheel or window	Suspect skull fractures (see page 69). Treat for concussion or compression, if present (see page 70)

CYCLISTS – MOTORCYCLISTS AND PUSH CYCLISTS

INJURY	CAUSED BY	TREATMENT
Broken collar bone	Caused by falling on outstretched arm	Immobilisation – using elevation sling (see page 76) or improvised bandages
Friction burns	Moving along gravel, tarmac or grass	Cool burn and cover (see pages 87–88)
Head injuries	Going over handlebars	Suspect skull fractures (see page 69). Treat for concussion or compression, if present (see page 70)
		Refer to page 100 for treatment of a casualty wearing a helmet
Neck injuries	Impact	Keep head still. Apply improvised collar, if appropriate (see page 72). Only remove helmet if the casualty has breathing difficulties (see page opposite)
Heat-stroke/heat exhaustion/Sunburn (most particularly push cyclists)	Inadequate protection against the sun. Not taking enough fluids while cycling	Cool down burns (see pages 87–88). Replace fluid if you suspect heat exhaustion (see page 96). Cool the casualty if you suspect heat-stroke (see page 96)

PEDESTRIANS

INJURY	CAUSED BY	TREATMENT
Fractures of the lower leg	Impact of bumper on shin	Immobilise legs (see page 77)
Head injuries	Hitting head on windshield after rolling across bonnet	Suspect skull fractures (see page 69). Treat for concussion or compression, if present (see page 70)

REMOVING A CRASH HELMET

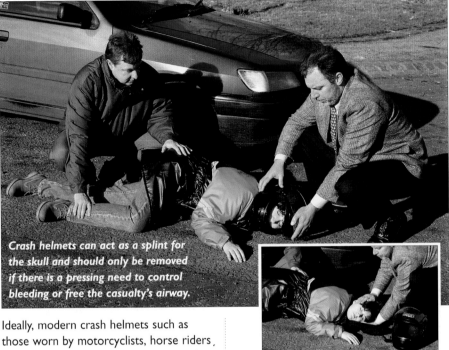

Crash helmets can act as a splint for the skull and should only be removed if there is a pressing need to control bleeding or free the casualty's airway.

Ideally, modern crash helmets such as those worn by motorcyclists, horse riders, and now increasingly push cyclists, are best left on the casualty.

These particular road users run a high risk of head and neck injuries because of the typically 'up and over' nature of the accidents that they may suffer. Removing a crash helmet increases the risk of further damage to the neck, and if there are head injuries the helmet may be acting as a splint holding the skull still.

The main reason for removing a helmet (see page 100 for the method) is if the casualty's airway is obstructed (by vomiting, blood or the helmet itself). You also need to remove the helmet if there is severe bleeding to the head which you cannot control without applying direct pressure.

MOTORCYCLE HELMETS

Many motorcycle helmets now come with a face plate that can be removed without taking off the rest of the helmet. This section is often released by pressing two buttons either side of the jaw.

In full-face helmets without this feature, you may find that opening the visor will allow you sufficient access to the casualty's airway or bleeding to avoid having to take off the entire helmet.

However, if there is no choice but to remove the helmet, this manoeuvre should be carried out by two people, as detailed on the next page.

STEP 1

Kneeling beside the casualty, the first aider should concentrate on the casualty's neck, gently easing their fingers under the helmet and supporting the neck and jaw by spreading out their fingers.

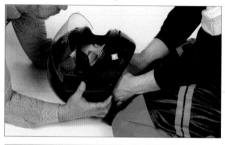

STEP 2

The helper should gently tilt the helmet (not the head) backwards and move the helmet over the nose and then over the rest of the head.

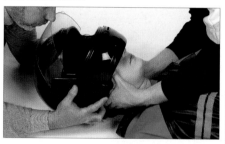

STEP 3

It is important that the person supporting the neck does not let go once the helmet has been removed. If they do the head will drop to the ground leading to potential neck damage.

STEP 4

Place a cushion carefully under the casualty's head and support the head with hands either side to tilt the jaw up to help maintain a clear airway.

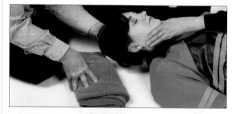

RIDING HAT AND PUSH-CYCLIST HELMETS

These rarely obstruct the face and airway, but if it is essential to remove them, unfasten or cut though the strap and gently ease the sides of the helmet out and away from the casualty's face. Then lift the helmet upwards and backwards off the head.

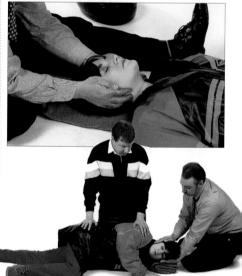

If the casualty needs to be placed in the recovery position, it is important to keep the head raised so that the spine is kept in a straight line.

Medical Conditions

THIS CHAPTER FOCUSES ON THOSE medical conditions which can become medical emergencies. While drivers do not run a higher risk than average of coming across these conditions, it is important for everyone to be able to recognise the signs and symptoms and to be able to carry out the simple but potentially life saving procedures as necessary.

Medical conditions covered in this chapter

- Asthma
- Heart attack
- Allergic reactions
- Stroke
- Angina
- Cardiac arrest
- Epilepsy

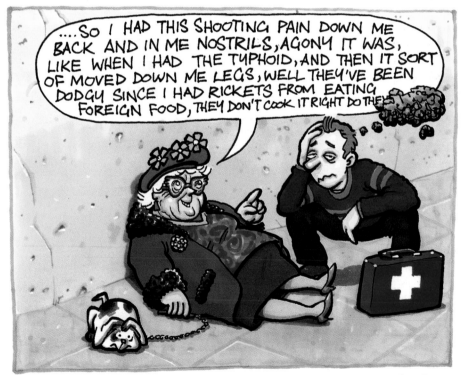

You won't be much use as a first aider to a casualty suffering from a condition other than an injury if you can't recognise the condition's signs and symptoms right away.

ASTHMA

Asthma appears to be increasing in its frequency. Most of us will know somebody who carries an inhaler for the prevention of asthma. Many of us may have family members, particularly children, who suffer from the condition.

WHAT IS IT?

Asthma attacks cause the muscles of the air passages to go into a spasm, making it very difficult for the sufferer to breathe.

Attacks may be triggered by an allergy or by stress – a friend of mine recently had a very bad attack triggered by her involvement in a car crash. The attacks are very distressing both for the sufferer and for those who are watching.

ASTHMA SIGNS AND SYMPTOMS

- **Difficulty in breathing, particularly breathing out**

- **Wheezing or otherwise noisy breathing**

- **Inability to speak**

- **Pale skin with potential cyanosis (blue skin, particularly around the lips)**

- **Distress, dizziness and confusion as it becomes harder to get oxygen into the body**

- **Potential unconsciousness and respiratory arrest.**

ASTHMA TREATMENT

Asthma should not be underestimated. While the preventative treatments are very effective and the drugs to relieve attacks are very effective, left untreated, a serious attack can be fatal. The strain of a serious asthma attack can cause respiratory failure or even cardiac arrest. The first aider should be prepared to resuscitate the casualty if necessary (see pages 39–47).

STEP 1

Reassure the casualty, as this will have a positive effect on their breathing.

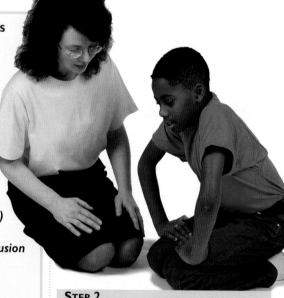

STEP 2

Help the casualty to sit or kneel leaning slightly forward, since most asthmatics find this an easier position for breathing.

STEP 3
If the casualty has medication, enable them to use it – inhalers are the main form of treatment and are generally blue-coloured.

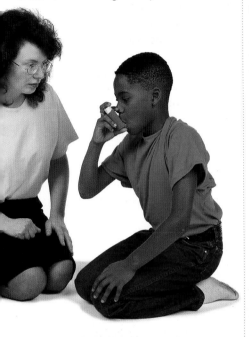

⚠️ IF THIS IS THE SUFFERER'S first attack, or the medication dose not work, or the casualty is in severe respiratory distress, **call an ambulance**. If the attack eases and the casualty finds it easier to breathe, they will not need immediate medical attention but should advise their doctor of the attack. They will often be very tired, so it is best to ensure that they are accompanied home.

HYPERVENTILATION

Another area of breathing difficulty which may be triggered by the stress of an accident is hyperventilation. Here, the casualty 'over breathes', unbalancing the amount of oxygen and carbon dioxide in the blood. It is this imbalance that leads to the signs and symptoms of fast and deep breathing, a feeling of pins and needles in the limbs, dizziness and cramps. While asthma is caused by a physical condition which may be triggered by a stressful experience, hyperventilation is generally caused by psychological stress.

HYPERVENTILATION TREATMENT

STEP 1
If the casualty is otherwise uninjured, remove them from the scene of the accident to a quiet place with no 'audience'.

STEP 2
Reassure the casualty, remain calm, speak firmly. Encourage them to regain control of their breathing. Do not slap the casualty.

STEP 3
If the condition persists, and you are certain there are no other underlying conditions, let the casualty breathe their own air from a paper bag. This helps to balance the ratio of oxygen and carbon dioxide in the blood.

STEP 4
Be prepared to call a doctor or an ambulance if the casualty's symptoms do not disappear.

ANGINA PECTORIS

Throughout life our arteries are clogging up with fatty deposits. The speed at which arteries are blocked is increased through a lack of exercise, a high fat diet, smoking and high stress levels. As these fatty deposits cause the coronary (heart) and other arteries to become narrower, it becomes increasingly difficult for blood to flow around the body.

Under normal circumstances, clogged coronary arteries can just about supply blood to the heart. But under the duress of emotional upset or sudden exercise the heart rate speeds up as the body demands more highly-oxygenated blood; and then the coronary arteries fail to cope with the demand. It is not uncommon for people to have angina attacks after being involved in a high-stress activity such as a road accident.

This leads to *angina pectoris*, which, literally translated, means 'crushing of the chest'. The pain is severe and very frightening, but acts as a warning to the casualty to calm down or to rest.

ANGINA SIGNS AND SYMPTOMS

- *Gripping chest pain, often described by the casualty as 'vicelike'*

- *This pain may radiate up into the jaw and/or down into the left arm*

- *There may be a feeling of pins and needles down the arm*

- *A shortness of breath*

- *Dizziness and confusion*

- *Anxiety*

- *Pale skin, with possible cyanosis*

- *A rapid weak pulse.*

ANGINA TREATMENT

STEP 1

Sit the casualty down and reassure them. This reduces the demands being placed on the heart.

STEP 2

Angina sufferers may have medication to relieve an attack, usually a puffer, or tablet which is placed under the tongue. The medication works by dilating the blood vessels, therefore increasing circulation to the heart muscle and around the body. Help the casualty to take this medication.

STEP 3

Call an ambulance if the pain does not appear to ease or if the casualty is not a known angina sufferer.

If the casualty has regular attacks listen to what they want to do next. They should not be left alone. They should advise their doctor of the attack.

HEART ATTACKS

If some of the coronary arteries become completely blocked, the area of the heart muscle being supplied by those blood vessels will be starved of oxygen and will eventually die. This blockage may be caused by a clot – a condition you may have heard referred to as a *coronary thrombosis*.

The effect of this blockage will depend on how big an area of the heart muscle is affected. If only a small area of the heart dies off, it is entirely possible for someone not to realise that they are having a heart attack – the little pain associated with this level of heart attack is often shrugged off as indigestion. Without treatment, smaller heart attacks are likely to continue over a period of months or years and eventually a large area of the heart will die. This leads to the heart stopping – cardiac arrest.

But it is not all doom and gloom. Anti-clotting medicines have proved very effective in the prevention of further heart attacks. They may even be given to high-risk patients to prevent an attack happening in the first place. Commonplace aspirin has also proved itself to have a place in coronary care as it thins the blood, which improves circulation.

The development of advanced cardiac in-hospital and good post-hospital care means that heart attack patients have a good chance of making a full recovery – important information to remember when you are reassuring a very distressed casualty.

The advent of the defibrillator has meant that even if a heart attack has led to a cardiac arrest, some patients still have a good chance of survival.

It is important to note that although the signs and symptoms are much the same as those of angina (see *page 104*) – indeed the patient may initially suffer an angina attack which becomes a heart attack – there are key differences, outlined below.

HEART ATTACK
SIGNS AND SYMPTOMS

■ *Feeling of indigestion and general discomfort for milder attacks*

■ *No recovery on rest. While angina sufferers will recover from their attack on resting, heart attack patients do not tend to improve without medical treatment*

■ *A feeling of impending doom – patients have described the sensation of feeling as if their bodies were aware of what was happening to them*

■ *Possible deterioration into unconsciousness, respiratory arrest or cardiac arrest*

■ *Angina attacks tend to come on after exercise or stress, while heart attacks do not necessarily follow exertion – indeed, one of the most common times for heart attacks to occur is while sleeping.*

The first aid treatment for heart attacks follows on page 106.

HEART ATTACK TREATMENT

STEP 1
Move the casualty into a half-sitting position; head and shoulders supported and knees bent, as this is generally the best position to breath in. Place a rolled-up blanket under the knees to support them.

STEP 2
Reassure the casualty and do not let them move as this will place an extra strain on the heart.

STEP 3
Call for an ambulance as soon as possible.

STEP 4
If the casualty has angina medication, allow them to take this. If you have an ordinary aspirin, allow them to chew one (without water).

STEP 5
Keep a continual check on the breathing and pulse, and be prepared to resuscitate, if necessary (see pages 39–47).

If the casualty is unconscious, place in the recovery position (see pages 23–25) and ensure they are kept warm.

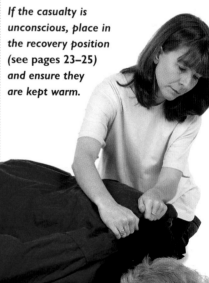

ALLERGIC REACTIONS

The number of people suffering allergic reactions appears to be on the increase. Perhaps people are becoming more sensitive to allergens (the substances that cause allergic reactions), or perhaps we are getting better at detecting allergies.

For the first aider, the biggest concern is anaphylactic shock – an extreme allergic reaction, which has intense effects on the body. Alarmingly, anaphylaxis can happen very quickly – within seconds. Anaphylactic shock can be caused by many substances, but the most common culprits are:

- nuts – for those who are particularly sensitive even touching the trace of a nut can be potentially fatal
- seafood
- insect stings and bites
- drugs – some people have a very extreme reaction to penicillin, for example.

ALLERGY SIGNS AND SYMPTOMS

One of the main effects of severe anaphylaxis is a dilation of the blood vessels and a constriction of the air passages (a similar condition to asthma, but generally more severe, preventing intake of any oxygen).

- *Difficulty in breathing*

- *Pale skin and cyanosis*

- *Blotchy patches on the skin*

- *A rapid pulse*

- *Respiratory or cardiac arrest*

- *History of contact to allergens – anaphylaxis happens very quickly.*

ALLERGIC REACTIONS TREATMENT

STEP 1
Call an ambulance immediately. The casualty needs an adrenaline injection to counteract the reaction.

STEP 2
If the casualty is a known sufferer, they may have an adrenaline injection. Assist them to give this. If they are unable – and you have been trained to do so – give them the injection yourself.

STEP 3
Sit the casualty in their most comfortable position and reassure them.

STEP 4
If the casualty goes unconscious, move them into the recovery position. Monitor breathing and circulation. Be ready to resuscitate if necessary.

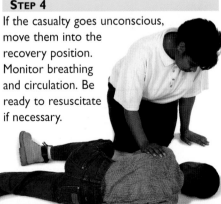

EPILEPSY

Epilepsy is a very common condition. It is best described as a rogue electrical discharge across the brain. As the body's functions are controlled by electrical impulses, this discharge can lead to a number of physical reactions.

Many things may trigger a fit. It is not unusual for a passenger in a car on bright days to have a fit triggered by the flashing light of the sun behind trees, or for a stressful situation to bring on a fit.

EPILEPSY TREATMENT

Step 1

During the fit do not attempt to restrain the casualty. While under the influence of the fit, the casualty will have no awareness of their actions, and the muscular contractions that take place during a fit are so strong that holding them down or restraining them in any way may lead to broken bones – yours and theirs.

DO NOT ATTEMPT to put anything in the mouth. An epileptic is unlikely to bite their tongue, but even if they do, it is unlikely to cause problems if they are treated correctly. Much more of a risk is broken teeth when a spoon has been forced into the mouth.

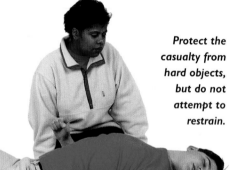

Protect the casualty from hard objects, but do not attempt to restrain.

Step 2

When the fit is over, check the casualty's airway and breathing, as you would with any unconscious person. Problems are rare, but choking may be an issue if they were eating something before the fit, and they may have suffered head injuries. Be prepared to carry out the procedures for choking or to resuscitate, if necessary.

Step 3

When the casualty comes round, reassure them. They may have wet or soiled themselves, so cover them up and then when they are steady on their feet, help them to find somewhere to clean up. They are likely to be very tired. If possible, find them somewhere to lie down and sleep. Ask them what they want to do – most epileptics manage their condition well and will have their own strategies for coping.

CALLING AN AMBULANCE

Generally epilepsy is not a medical emergency. However, you should be prepared to call an ambulance if:

- the casualty injures themselves during the fit
- the fit lasts for longer than five minutes
- the casualty has repeated fits in a short period of time
- the casualty does not regain consciousness.

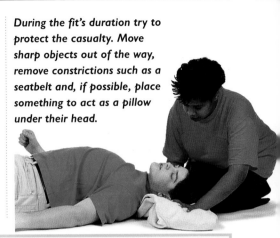

During the fit's duration try to protect the casualty. Move sharp objects out of the way, remove constrictions such as a seatbelt and, if possible, place something to act as a pillow under their head.

TYPES OF EPILEPTIC FITS

ABSENCES – MINOR FITS

During minor epilepsy, the casualty suffers a brief disturbance in the brain's normal activity, leading to a lack of awareness of their surroundings. To the observer, it might seem like they are daydreaming or that they have suddenly switched off.

There is little for the first aider to do other than to guide the casualty away from danger and reassure them when they come back to their normal state. If they have not been aware of any similar fits before, advise them to see their doctor.

MAJOR FITS

This is what most people would recognise as epilepsy. There are typically four stages to this fit.

1. Many people get an aura that a fit is likely to occur. While this generally immediately precedes the fit, an ex-colleague of mine could smell bananas some 20 minutes before the fit occurred and could get himself lying down comfortably in a safe position.

2. The electrical impulses lead to a contraction in the muscles. The casualty will often fall to the ground with a cry as the contraction of the respiratory muscles forces the air out of the lungs and leaves the muscles rigid. This is known as the *tonic* phase. The casualty's muscles may then go into spasm known as the *clonic* phase. During this stage the casualty will not be breathing.

3. When the fit is finished the casualty will be in a state of unconsciousness.

4. On recovering consciousness the casualty will be very sleepy.

STROKE

A stroke is caused either by a blood clot in the arteries supplying the brain or a burst blood vessel. Both situations will lead to a reduction in blood flow and the eventual death of that area of the brain.

The signs and symptoms are similar to those of compression (*see page 70*). The extent of the effect of the stroke will depend on how much of the brain has died and which areas are affected. Different parts of the brain control different functions. If the stroke has affected the area of the brain controlling speech, the casualty might have difficulty talking; speech may be slurred and difficult to understand.

As with heart attacks, the degree of the stroke can vary greatly. If the stroke is small, the casualty may not even realise that they have suffered one as the signs and symptoms may only include a headache or slight dizziness.

STROKE SIGNS AND SYMPTOMS

- *Headache and/or dizziness*

- *Confusion*

- *Slurred speech*

- *Flushed face*

- *Slow and full pulse*

- *Noisy breathing*

- *Paralysis or difficulty in moving one side of the body*

- *Possible unconsciousness*

- *Respiratory and cardiac arrest*

STROKE TREATMENT

STEP 1

Sit the casualty up and make them comfortable. They are likely to be confused and frustrated because they may not be able to make themselves understood. Be patient with them and set up a simple method of communication.

STEP 2

Call an ambulance. If the casualty becomes unconscious, place them into the recovery position and monitor the breathing and circulation. Be prepared to resuscitate, if necessary (*see pages 39–47*).

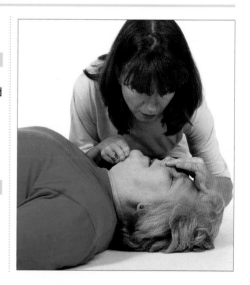

Emergency Index

WHILE IT IS VITAL THAT YOU READ the contents of this book to gain more detailed knowledge, *First Aid for Motorists*' EMERGENCY INDEX will enable you to find the key information that you will require at a glance.

And once you have become proficient in the subject of first aid, the EMERGENCY INDEX on the following pages will also act as a refresher to the key steps in most emergency cases you are likely to encounter. However, the briefly stated points in the index should be taken in conjunction with the detailed contents of the main body of this book. (*Red numbers* in the text refer to page numbers.)

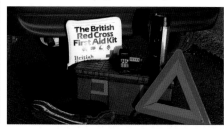

INDEX CONTENTS

APPROACHING AN ACCIDENT SCENE

IMPORTANT POINTS TO REMEMBER

Do not rush.

If you are in a car, ensure that you check mirrors and pull over safely.

Pull up behind the incident to protect the scene from oncoming drivers.

Ensure that you and your car are visible.

If you use hazard lights, only apply them when you are stationary.

Set up the hazard warning triangle to alert oncoming drivers. If it is safe to do so, enlist the help of a bystander to flag down approaching traffic.

If it is dark, wear light-coloured clothing in order to be seen by approaching traffic.

Check for danger.

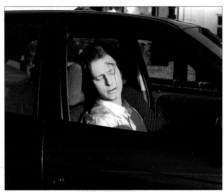

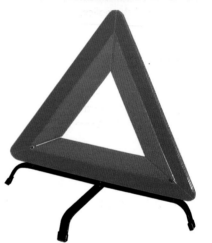

REDUCING FIRE RISK

Ensure nobody smokes around the accident site.

Ensure the ignition of any involved vehicle is switched off.

Isolate the batteries of any vehicles involved in the accident.

Cover petrol spills with earth, and keep bystanders away from the accident.

Do not attempt to rescue people trapped in a burning car.

Call the fire brigade, and get everybody back from the accident scene.

Do not attempt to fight the fire yourself.

ARRANGING FOR HELP

ASSESS THE ACCIDENT

Determine which casualties are most in need of urgent attention.

Remember that the quietest casualties are probably the ones whose lives are most in danger from their injuries.

DIAL 999

If in doubt about which emergency services you require, call the police who will contact the appropriate help.

Give your name and the number you are calling from.

Describe the location of the accident precisely – identify landmarks, junction numbers and house numbers in a residential area.

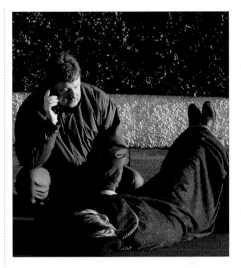

Describe the nature of the accident, inluding any hazards, trapped casualties, number of casualties, types of injury.

Do not hang up until the operator tells you to.

FIRST AID KIT

Disposable gloves.

Triangular bandages.

Large sterile dressing.

Plasters for smaller cuts and grazes.

Alcohol-free wipes to clean small wounds.

Sandwich bags for enclosing burns.

Safety pins for fastening bandages.

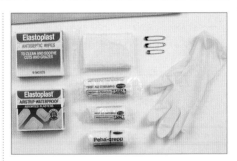

Pair of round-nosed scissors.

Water.

Kits are available from your local British Red Cross branch.

BSM

RESUSCITATION SEQUENCE

1 Check for danger. Then follow these general procedures (39–47)

2 Assess the casualty's condition. Open the casualty's airway.

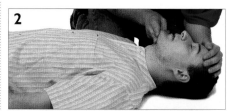

3 Check the casualty's breathing.

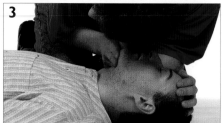

4 If breathing, turn the casualty into the recovery position.

5 If not breathing, give the casualty two artificial ventilations, inflating for approximately two seconds.

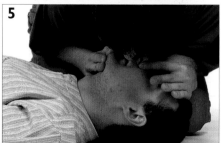

6 Check the casualty's circulation for up to ten seconds.

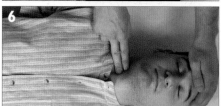

7 If circulation is present, continue with ventilations, rechecking the circulation every ten breaths.

8 If circulation is absent, alternate 15 chest compressions, at a rate of 100 a minute and a depth of 4–5 cms, with two ventilations.

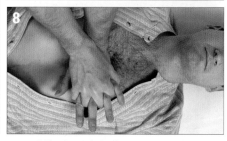

Call an ambulance at the earliest appropriate opportunity.

✱ Numbers in red refer to main entries in the book

UNCONSCIOUS CASUALTIES

ASSESSING CASUALTIES, CLEARING THE AIRWAY

1 Check for danger. This remains your priority even if you suspect that one or more of the casualties is unconscious.

2 Assess the condition of the casualties.
The quietest casualty is often the one who is most at risk.

3

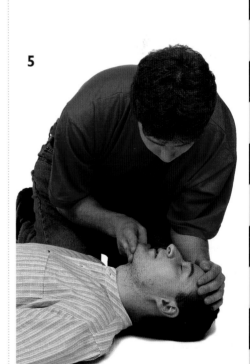

3 Check to see if the casualty is really unconscious. Kneel down next to the casualty and ask them a question to try and provoke a response. If this fails, shake the casualty by the shoulders (be gentle as there may be the risk of neck injuries). If there is still no response, assume that the casualty is unconscious.

5

4 Clear the casualty's airway by removing potential obstructions to breathing. If this is not possible, call for help immediately.

5 Prevent the casualty from choking on their tongue by opening the airway.
Place two fingers under the chin and lift the jaw. Place your other hand on the forehead and gently tilt the head backwards. This will stop the tongue from resting on the back of the throat and will maintain an open airway (*21, 39*)

❋ *Numbers in red refer to main entries in the book*

CHECKING BREATHING

1 Look. Maintain the lifted jaw and tilted head position. Look to see if the chest is rising and falling.

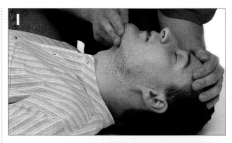

2 Listen for the sounds of breathing with your cheek by the side of the casualty's mouth.

3 Feel the casualty's breaths on your cheek (22, 39)

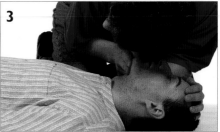

4 If breathing, place in the recovery position (23–25)

CHECKING CIRCULATION

1 Check the casualty's circulation. Take the pulse at the neck – at the carotid artery. If there is no pulse, commence CPR (39–47)

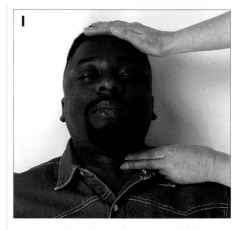

2 If there is a pulse, record its strength and the rhythm.

3 Keep checking every five minutes and pass the information to the ambulance service.

4 If the pulse becomes quick and gets weaker, suspect shock. Check for any external bleeding, and treat the casualty for shock (50–52)

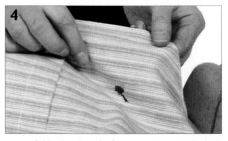

■ The average adult pulse rate is between 60 and 80 heart beats per minute (children and infants have a slightly faster pulse).

❋ *Numbers in red refer to main entries in the book*

RECOVERY POSITION

1 Ensure the jaw is lifted and the head is back. Place the arm nearest you underneath the body, fingers flat, palm upwards, elbow straight.

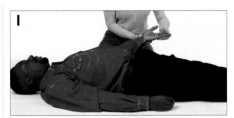

2 Bring the arm furthest from you over the casualty's chest. Hold the hand at the face palm outwards.

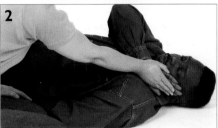

3 With your other hand, bend the leg furthest from you just above the knee and place the foot flat on the floor.

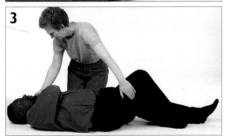

4 Supporting the hand at the face and placing a hand on the leg, move the casualty towards you until the knee touches the ground. Use your knees to prevent the casualty slipping too far forward.

5 Ensure that the head is tilted back. If necessary, place their hand under the face. Adjust the positioning of the leg so that the casualty is stable and will not move any further.

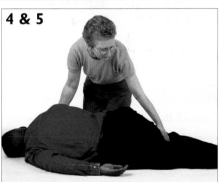

6 Maintain a check on the casualty's breathing and circulation and ensure than an ambulance has been called (23–25)

❋ Numbers in red refer to main entries in the book

SPINAL INJURY RECOVERY POSITION

This manoeuvre requires at least two people. If you have been trained to do so, move the head into the neutral position, if it is not already there (26–27)

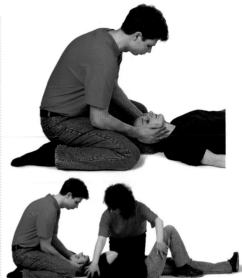

1 Support the head, firmly placing your hands over the casualty's ears. You must keep the head in line with the neck and spine and reduce the movement of the head from side to side.

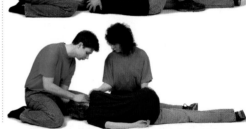

2 The second person prepares for the recovery position as shown on the opposite page.

3 Move the casualty slowly over onto their side, keeping the head in line with the body.

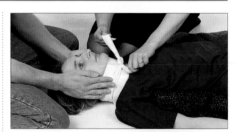

4 Continue to support the head when the casualty is on their side. If possible, the second first aider should continue to support the body.

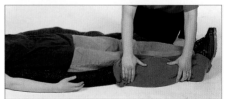

ADDITIONAL SUPPORT

If you suspect a neck injury, a collar can be applied for additional support.

If the casualty has fractures, ensure that the fracture is supported when turning into the recovery position. Keep broken arms and legs straight, and use rolled up coats or blankets as props to ensure that the casualty stays on their side.

✳ *Numbers in red refer to main entries in the book*

HOW TO GIVE ARTIFICIAL VENTILATIONS

1 Remove obstructions from the mouth. Extended head and lift jaw. Pinch the casualty's nose shut.

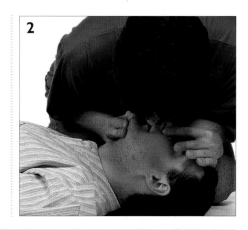

2 Place your lips around the casualty's mouth and breathe into the casualty's airway, taking approximately two seconds to inflate their lungs.

3 Take your mouth away from the casualty's mouth and watch the chest drop. Repeat the procedure, giving the casualty two breaths in total (40)

HOW TO GIVE CHEST COMPRESSIONS

ADULTS

Place the heel of your hand on the lower half of the sternum. Place your other hand on top and interlock the fingers, pulling them off the chest. Lock your elbows straight and push down, compressing the chest 4–5 cm at a rate of 100 a minute (42–43)

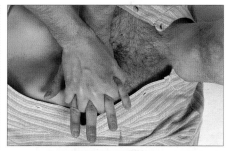

CHILDREN

Place the heel of your hand on the lower half of the breast bone and compress to a third of the depth of the chest at a rate of 100 a minute (45)

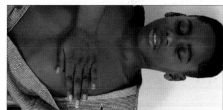

INFANTS

Holding the infant, place two fingers on the lower half of the breast bone. Compress to a third of the depth of the chest at the rate of 100 a minute (47)

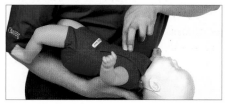

✱ Numbers in red refer to main entries in the book

CHOKING ADULT

CONSCIOUS

1 Encourage the casualty to cough.

2 If coughing is ineffective, lean the casualty forward and hit firmly between their shoulder blades, up to five sharp slaps.

3 If this does not work, use up to five abdominal thrusts.

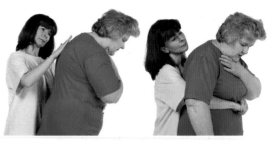

4 Alternate back slaps with abdominal thrusts until the object is cleared. If the object does not come up, ensure that an ambulance has been called (32)

UNCONSCIOUS

1 Open the airway and assess breathing.

2 If the casualty is not breathing, attempt artificial ventilations.

3 If unable to ventilate, turn the casualty onto their side and give up to five sharp blows between the shoulder blades. Check the mouth and remove any loose objects.

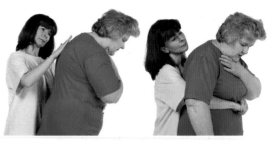

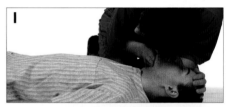

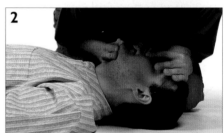

4 If back slaps fail, place the heel of your hand below their ribcage and press sharply up towards the diaphragm.

5 If the casualty is still not breathing, ensure that an ambulance has been called. Attempt to ventilate again. If you still cannot get air in, repeat steps 3 and 4 until either the ambulance arrives or the casualty starts to breathe (33)

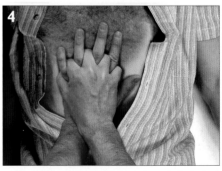

✳ *Numbers in red refer to main entries in the book*

CHOKING CHILD

CONSCIOUS

1 Bend the child over your lap, head lower than chest. Hit on the back up to five times, with a flat hand. Check mouth and remove any obstruction after every step.

2 If this does not work, use up to five chest thrusts at a rate of one thrust every three seconds.

3 If step 2 does not work, use abdominal thrusts.

4 If child is still choking, call an ambulance. Repeat steps 1–3 until help arrives or the obstruction clears (*34*)

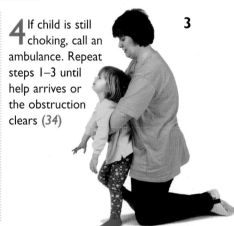

3

UNCONSCIOUS

1 Open airway, using head tilt and jaw lift, and assess breathing. If they are not breathing, attempt artificial ventilations.

2 If you cannot ventilate, turn the casualty onto their side and give up to five back slaps. Then repeat step 1.

3 If you still cannot ventilate, turn face upwards on the floor and give up to five chest compressions. Repeat step 1.

4 If you still cannot ventilate, give up to five abdominal thrusts. Repeat step 1.

5 Call for an ambulance, and repeat steps 2–4 until help arrives (*35*)

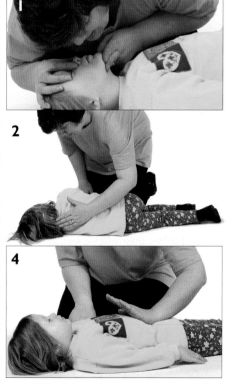

✻ *Numbers in red refer to main entries in the book*

CHOKING INFANT

1 Lay a conscious infant face down on your forearm, supporting the neck and head. Give up to five slaps on the back.

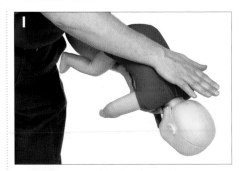

2 Check the casualty's mouth, and gently remove any obvious obstructions with one finger.

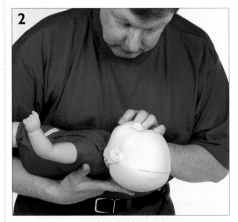

3 If this has not cleared the obstruction, turn the casualty over so that they are lying face up along your arm (or lay them on your lap), with the head supported. Using two fingers, give up to five chest compressions. Repeat step 2.

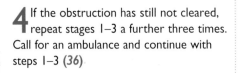

4 If the obstruction has still not cleared, repeat stages 1–3 a further three times. Call for an ambulance and continue with steps 1–3 (36)

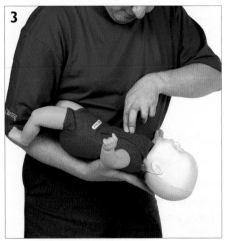

DO NOT feel down an infant's throat.

DO NOT use abdominal thrusts on an infant; resuscitate if necessary.

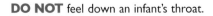
✸ Numbers in red refer to main entries in the book

BLEEDING

EXTERNAL WOUNDS

1 Check extent of wound. Look for secondary areas of bleeding. Check there are no foreign bodies in the wound.

2 Apply pressure to the wound with your fingers over a sterile dressing.

3 Apply a fresh sterile dressing held in place with a firm bandage.

4 On limbs, elevate the wound above the level of the heart.

5 Treat the casualty for shock, sitting or lying them down. Keep them warm.

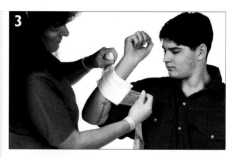

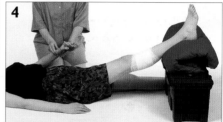

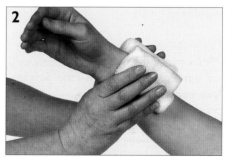

FOREIGN BODIES

1 Do not remove the object. Apply pressure around wound edges without pressing on the foreign object (58–59)

2 Using clean pads, build a bridge either side of the wound to protect it. Then bandage firmly in place.

3 Elevate injured limbs if possible.

4 Treat for shock (50–52)

Prevent longer objects from moving by supporting them with your hands or by packing a coat around the base of the object.

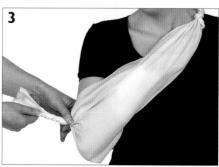

✷ *Numbers in red refer to main entries in the book*

FRACTURES

GENERAL TREATMENT

Keep the casualty still. If need be, help the casualty into a comfortable position. Help steady and support the fracture using your hands. If you have to transport the casualty yourself, or if it is going to be a while until help arrives, immobilise the fracture further with bandages or by improvising with coats, blankets, etc. But remember not to tie the bandage too tightly and to pad around the site of the fracture.

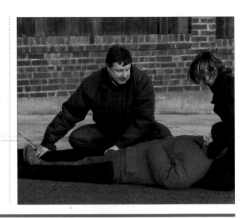

SKULL FRACTURES

Keep the casualty still while they are conscious. Keep a check on their ABC. Resuscitate or turn into recovery position, if necessary. Call for medical aid as soon as possible.

If there is fluid coming from the ear, place this ear downwards and cover it with a sterile pad. But do not plug the pad into the ear.

With fractures to the bones of the face and jaw ensure that any blood in the mouth is allowed to dribble out. Gently

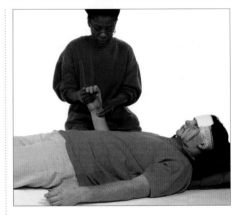

remove any teeth or bits of broken bone from the mouth. Get the casualty to hospital as soon as possible (69)

TREATING CONCUSSION

1 Place in recovery position, if necessary, and monitor ABC (70).

2 Call an ambulance if the casualty does not recover after three minutes or if there are signs of skull fracture or compression.

TREATING COMPRESSION

1 If unconscious, place the casualty in the recovery position and monitor ABC. If conscious, lay the casualty down with their head and shoulders slightly raised (70)

2 Maintain a close check on the ABC. Call an ambulance as soon as possible.

✱ Numbers in red refer to main entries in the book

SPINAL FRACTURES

CONSCIOUS

1 Casualties still in their car should be left there. Ensure that an ambulance has been called. Hold the casualty's head still (**72**)

2 If you have a long wait for the ambulance, and the injury is to the neck, ask a bystander to improvise a neck collar (*right*). Maintain head support after the collar has been applied.

UNCONSCIOUS

1 ABC is first priority. Take care to tilt the head gently. If the casualty is not breathing, resuscitate. To place on their back, keep the head, trunk and toes in a straight line (**73**)

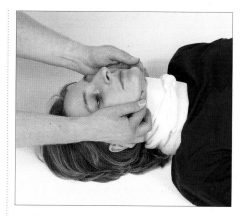

2 If they are breathing and on their side, head extended, leave them there. Hold the head as for conscious casualties. Monitor the airway.

3 If the head is not extended or they are not on their side, move them into the spinal injury recovery position. (**26–27**)

LONG BONE FRACTURES

To immobilise a broken arm, use a triangular bandage, or similar, to improvise an arm sling (**75**)

For fractures to the hand or collar bone, use an elevation sling (**76**)

With fractures of the legs, hold the injured part still and treat the casualty for shock. Support leg above and below the fracture with your hands or by placing padding around the broken leg (**77**). Only employ traction if you have been trained to do so.

MULTIPLE RIB FRACTURES

Lay conscious casualties down or have them half-sitting. Lean the casualty towards their injured side. Treat sucking wounds. Treat any open fractures. Place the arm on the injured side into an elevation sling (**76**) Treat the casualty for shock.

With unconscious casualties, monitor their ABC and place them into the recovery position with their injured side upwards.

❋ *Numbers in red refer to main entries in the book*

BURGS

GENERAL TREATMENT

1 Protect yourself. Ensure that fires are out, electrical equipment is disconnected and chemical spills will not affect you.

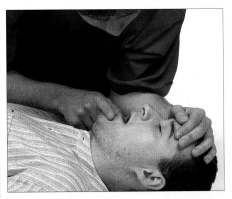

2 Check the casualty's ABC. Douse burnt area with cool liquid to reduce pain, swelling and risk of scarring. Avoid over-cooling, restrict liquid to the injured part. DO NOT apply water under pressure.

3 Assess whether or not an ambulance is needed. Keep cooling injured part until pain stops. Cover wound with a sterile bandage tied loosely over the burn. Elevate the injured part using an elevation sling (76)

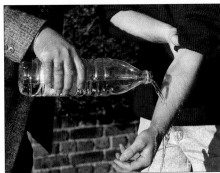

4 Treat for shock. Monitor ABC. Check that bandages are not too tight as the wounded area begins to swell.

DO NOT put fluffy material, creams or ointments on the burn. Do not burst blisters, or remove burnt clothing which may be sticking to the wound.

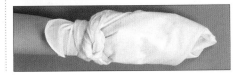

CHEMICAL BURNS

Refer to HAZCHEM symbols (16) and call for professional help (inform the ambulance service it is a chemical burn). Wear protective clothing. Ventilate enclosed areas. Make sure contaminated cooling water runs away from you and the casualty. If possible, remove contaminated clothes from the casualty without harming yourself.

ELECTRICAL BURNS

Do not touch the casualty if they are in contact with live equipment. Turn off the electricity at the mains point or move the casualty from the contact using a non-conducting material. A casualty suffering from an electrical burn may well have respiratory or circulatory difficulties, so resuscitation may be necessary.

✱ Numbers in red refer to main entries in the book

Details of the royalties payable to the British Red Cross Society, a registered charity, can be obtained by writing to the publisher.